SINS

OF

NURSES

FIRST EDITION www.sinsofnurses.com

The Nursing homes phone is ringing. Callers holding on the line here this. " Thanks for calling Golden and Great Nursing and Rehab, your call is important to us so please don't hang up. Here at Golden and Great Nursing and Rehab, your loved one is very important to us. Their health, safety and well being is also important to us. (Please don't hang up, someone will be with you shortly) Here at "Golden and Great Nursing and Rehab" we have plenty to keep our residents busy. We've enlisted the help of dozens of volunteers to assist wherever a bit of extra TLC is needed; for those times when you can't be here. We have a beautiful garden where residents are encouraged to cultivate and maintain former enjoyed past times. We have computer learning hour to keep the mind pliable and in touch with things locally and around the world. We even have cooking and baking hour "mmmm cookies." We have a projector tv room where residents may watch their favorite old movies at any hour of the day. There are daily scheduled activities in which your loved one may partake to keep away boredom... arts and crafts, bingo, board games, and of course therapy. Our Rehab Department is top notch, we leave no stone unturned. We will have your loved one walking and talking before you know it. We also have a memory care unit where we provide stimulating activities and a safe, secure environment to protect your loved one from harm.

In the meantime, I've been here for fourteen months and I have not seen one volunteer. If you aren't there to visit your loved one and to give that extra bit of TLC..."oh well." Anyway, that garden they mentioned is so over grown that you can't walk through it...no gardening being done there,ever... no flowers, just weeds, and dirt. This building holds over 200 residents and there are only two computers and one of them is broken. Good luck finding anyone to take your loved one to that one computer to keep their mind "pliable." As for that kitchen ,flat out, it is a staged none working area that gets no use. The projector TV room, well the tv is on but it's not playing any old movie. Its blaring with the lastest twerk music video. Young women half naked, dancing seductively. The daily activities usually include some form of music...probably rock and rap. Daily scheduled activities are a joke. Month after month, the same thing. Coffee time. Coloring. Maybe a board game, Bingo. Always Bingo. Church service. Usually while any of these activities is going on, you'll probably see ¾ of everyone there falling asleep. The Rehab/therapy department? Hard to get individuals who haven't talked in months or years to start talking again, individuals who have not walked in years, who have been in bed for months or even years, who are contracted Walking again, hell try getting someone like that to even sit up in the bed, or a wheelchair. Good luck with that walking and talking "thing." And Memory care aka locked away unit and that's that, locked away, can't get out, don't go past go! Your memory is gone. Welcome to Golden and Great Nursing and Rehab.

UNTOLD -TRUE ACCOUNTS-STORIES OF NURSING IN NURSING HOMES WRITTEN BY A NURSE. Nurses, do you wonder if nurses in Asia, Switzerland, Brazil, Germany, Africa, or even Idaho...anywhere/somewhere in the world experience the same challenges that U.S nurses deal with on a daily basis? This book tells stories of some of the things that we have to do, deal with, and accept as our realities on a daily basis. These are the things that happen when families leave and the doors shut.

"I have never met such cut-throat, back-stabbing, and unstable women in all my life." ##nurses

-Trina Macklin RN

ACKNOWLEDGEMENTS

THANK YOU TO GOD WHO GAVE ME THE STRENGTH, WISDOM, AND KNOWLEDGE TO WRITE THIS BOOK.

TO MY CHILDREN (AND GRANDCHILDREN), I LOVE YOU! THANK YOU TO MY RIDE OR DIE BESTIES WHO HELPED TO MAKE THIS BOOK POSSIBLE. YOU GUYS KNOW WHO YOU ARE.

A SPECIAL ACKNOWLEDGEMENT TO MAXINE N. MY FRIEND FOR OVER 15 YEARS. THANKS FOR ENCOURAGING ME, FRUSTRATING ME, AND ANNOYING ME ALONG THIS JOURNEY.

A SPECIAL THANK YOU TO MY CHILDHOOD PASTOR AND MAN OF GOD THE RIGHT REV. JOHN T. BETTS WHO IS GONE BUT NOT FORGOTTEN. MAY YOU KNOW HOW FAR YOUR TEACHINGS HAVE TAKEN ME THROUGHOUT MY LIFE?

FINALLY, TO MY FATHER, I MISS YOU, AND I KNOW YOU WOULD BE VERY PROUD OF THIS ACCOMPLISHMENT.

"There is no greater agony than bearing an untold story inside of you."

-Maya Angelou

INTRODUCTION

I've always wanted to go back to school to become a Registered Nurse (RN). It always seemed as if there would be plenty of time; then, there never seemed to be ENOUGH time or even a GOOD time. I am an Army trained licensed Practical Nurse (LPN); and from the minute that I entered nursing school and until the day that it was completed I knew that I wanted to experience every form of nursing that I could; and after I left the army, it felt natural for me to do just that. I guess being an RN just wasn't in the cards for me. So, I explored job opportunities that would allow me to explore nursing more fully. I was fortunate enough to have lived and worked as a nurse in many states (8 to be exact) and many cities within each state. I applied for any and every job that was of interest to me!

I applied, i interviewed and I always got the job. It seemed as though employers could since my training and know that I was a good nurse and I WAS! I was then and still am a fantastic nurse. I've worked in clinics (GI, GU, Pediatrics, Family Practice, Gyn, Internal Medicine), Private Duty (Adults and Pediatrics), Hospital (Departments of Pediatrics, Oncology, OB/GYN, Orthopedics and Emergency room), Home Health visits, Insurance company physicals, Correctional Nursing ,Interventional Radiology, Managed care projects, Insurance Audits ,Operating room Scrub and Circulator Tech, Mental health projects and last AND least the NURSING HOME.

I was and have always been full of pride in every job that I have ever taken. That was, until I started working in Nursing Homes. For all of my travels from state to state, it is known that an LPN can always find a job in a Nursing home. No matter the state, the city, the town, Nursing Homes are present; and tend to be the same. The similarities are overwhelmingly consistent. It's been a frustrating journey.

So, we nurses have to protect our licenses, we realize that we must remove medicine at its appropriate time.

I write this book with shame and a heavy heart for us all. It finally must be done. This book is not perfect, it's got it's grammatical flaws, sentence structure flaws, the flow may be off at times.

Try not to let those things distract you from the meaning and purpose of this book. Many stories are my own accounts , others shared/confided to me by other nurses and/or nursing assistants, some simply observed from the corners of my eyes, but all are the stories of RNs, LPNs and Nursing Assistants who work in a nursing home.

ALL ARE TRUE!!

I purposely do not and will not divulge which stories are my own and which were confided to me. This is for the safety of myself and those individuals. I've been collecting and writing these stories for over 20 years. I couldn't, if I wanted to give the names of the Nurses and CNA's whom some knowingly, others unknowingly contributed to the writing of this book. Just know that it is a compilation of stories that cover the everyday things that we do and encounter. Think of it as a bird's eye view into the daily world of the nursing home nurse. I think every nurse working in a nursing home will relate to these stories in SOME way. How much you relate to the stories as a Nurse or CNA will be based on how long you've been working in a nursing home. A person who has been a nurse or CNA for two years versus one who has been in this profession for 15 years will have different perspectives. Some of us will shake our heads in agreement and commonality, some stories will anger you, some may bore you, some may make you laugh and some stories may make you cry. They are my experiences, my truths..........These stories, for some, simply confirm that you are not alone. It's our way, my way of asking for forgiveness for a system that (I) we did not create and cannot control. I can only hope that after reading this book owners of Nursing Homes will work at making each of their facilities a better place for their patients and staff. One building at a time. Here's a suggestion if you really want to be make a change; hire a nurse, send them into your building, and ask for an honest account of their findings. They are not to divulge to anyone, not the managers, directors or even the administrators, who they are. They are to report to only you. Give it a week or two so that you get an accurate account. You will then know what kind of facility that you own. I assure you that you will be quite shocked at your report and if you care enough for people over money, which I doubt, then you will thank me. If you don't care to really know, then continue business as usual. These are my stories.

***SINS OF NURSES ***

SINS

OF

NURSES

TABLE OF CONTENTS

cleaning poop the next and then still the next minute calling a doctor for some other issue; after all, you are the supervisor. I must always deal with staffing issues because we are always short-staffed. For instance, if you were supposed to have 6 CNAs for today and only 4 showed up to work because two CNAs have called off, then the schedule has to be adjusted accordingly. This will then usually create a heavy workload for the staff that is there. This could mean that a CNA might have 15 residents that she or he is responsible for instead of the typical eight residents that she is responsible for. If a CNA has five residents out of her 10 that are total care and/or need lots of help, she will have to ask the nurse to help her. A nurse in a nursing home gets stretched a whole lot further than if she worked anywhere else, but then she usually gets paid more than if she worked anywhere else. The usual guideline regarding the medication pass is that a resident may receive their medication up to 1 hour before it's due and as late as 1 hour past its scheduled time. Therefore, medicine due at 9am may be given as early as 8am or as late as 10am. This formula sets the guideline for administering medication in skilled nursing facilities. If medicine cannot be given in this period, then it suggests that there might be a need for another nurse. For instance, 2 nurses passing medication for 9am, start at 7:30am, and finish around 10:30 or 11am. This would suggest that there is a need for three nurses. Most facilities are aware of this, but they continue to approve or turn a blind eye to what is substandard. They will leave the two nurses struggling daily. A nurse might have anywhere from 20-40 patients on a day shift. As for a night shift, don't ask! Imagine if you have 25 patients, and 12 of those patients are confused, five have g-tubes, and eight are alert and reasonably healthy. You have 2 hours to pass your "meds" or to do "pill call." A typical day might start something like this…arrive around 7 am, receive report (that's the report of what has happened with patients since you last worked), and do "rounds" (walk and check on your patients, making sure that everyone is in a stable condition). All of this usually takes about 30 minutes. Nevertheless, keep in mind that if the nurse that you are relieving leaves something unfinished from her shift, it becomes work that should be finished by YOU on YOUR shift. Not until report is over and you have keys in hand are all residents officially yours. I find that Nurses have really become inconsiderate when it comes to giving report. You can arrive on time, let the nurse you are relieving know that you are there, sit patiently and wait for report and keys. Nurses in 2018 will ignore you! This is fine by me; however, the problem becomes a problem when your shift starts at 7am. You are there at 6:55am. The nurse that you are relieving is walking around, being social, laughing, and talking about non-nursing things. You are waiting patiently. 07:20am, a resident falls.

FYI, don't look at me for help.

That incident report is ALL YOURS!!

FYI, KEEP HOLDING THE KEYS AND NOT GIVING REPORT.

Now you want to give report and count, and I'm a bitch because I'm not taking ownership of your incident report. "Have a great day." My shift has begun. Yours ended with a fall.

A typical shift starts with the inspection of the medication cart. You would typically look into the medication cart to make sure that you have everything that you need to get your day started. Usually, you don't have everything that you need! But then this will depend on the kind of facility that you work for. Some nursing homes have everything you need, and still, others have only the most minimal tools to do the job. Going forward, you are checking your cart for what you will need for the day. Checking for specific medications, bulk medicines, and usually a host of nutritional supplements. Many physicians want many of the residents to have these dietary supplements, about 60-120cc, depending on their dietary needs.

"YEAHHH!"

and on top of giving this supplement you must (you will try)to observe the resident until all of the medicine and supplement have been completed.

Try doing this before you move on to your next resident. Where has the time gone? It's now about 8am. Let's get started. Most days, you are overwhelmed before you have

Chapter 2

SOME THINGS DON'T CHANGE

I was sitting at the Nurses' desk when one of the CNAs rolled a wheelchair next to me, right in my line of sight, the resident looking dead at me. I know the CNA sat her there just to annoy me. "*Thanks,*" I thought to myself. "I'm going to leave Mrs. Langford here so that I can take care of one of my other patients, keep an eye on her for me.... please, and thank you." The nursing assistant said this with a smirk on her face as she hurried away. She knew very well that Mrs. Langford was going to disrupt everything and everyone around her while she sat at the nurses' station.

"Jessica!" I called, hoping that she would come back. She pretended not to hear me and kept walking. I hate it when the nursing assistants leave a resident at the nurses' station for the nurse to watch. Especially a resident like Mrs. Langford. They know that she is going to yell, scream, and bring havoc. "This is going to be an even longer day," I said aloud to no one in particular.

The morning had already been chaotic. I had a resident fall in the shower. I sent another one to the hospital, and my unit manager tells me that I have the joy of an admission coming before my shift will end. I look over at the clock. My shift ends in an hour, and I know I'm going to be here at least 2 hours beyond that.

Mrs. Langford has been a resident of our Nursing home for more than 10 years. She has multiple medical problems. But of all things to be concerned with, it is her advanced case of Dementia that has attributed to her being a problematic type of patient. "Why am I always getting the difficult patients on my assignment? Ugggh" If I take away the problematic side of dealing with Mrs. Langford, she is actually quite interesting. How can I describe her? Let's start with her education. It is well known that she was an educator, holds many degrees, and has taught several languages. Her resume is actually quite impressive. I'm told that she traveled around the world and lectured for many years. But, I believe that of all the things that she has done in her life, her studies of Greek and the Latin language are the most notable. She speaks fluent Latin most of the time, although she can speak English just as fluently. I'm not sure why she chooses to speak Latin more than she does English, I suppose it could be her dementia or maybe speaking Latin is the result of a longtime love for the language. With

where she wanted to be. Mary returned just in
can take her there, Nurse," says Mary.
gan to wheel her down the hall to her room. Just as
doing this, Mrs. Langford began to scream and

rs, Niggers, Niggers everywhere!!!"
r CNA called to Mary for help. She called to me.
can you take her to her room, I've got to help
Mrs. Langford continued to scream,
r nigger nigger!"
E HER!" I yelled, irritated.
isappeared into one of the rooms. I hurried down
toward her. I grabbed the wheelchair and paced
is I pushed her chair down the hall to her room. We
at her room; I pushed her inside and turned to walk
he whispered something. I turned and looked at
seemed to smirk at me, and then she yelled:
BYE, GET OUT NIGGER." I stared at her. Before I
iink, I SLAPPED HER!
your nigger!"
d out of her room with tears in my eyes.
he...Breathe......Take a deep breath., I didn't look back.

*** Sins of Nurses***

dementia patients, you never know why they do the things that they do. I don't know, and it's just as well that I don't spend any energy on the why of dementia, I have lots of other things that I could concern myself with.

There she sat at the nurses' station. Her 90lb tiny frame sitting in the wheelchair with her pale skin and very white naturally curly hair pulled on top of her head in a ragged bun. Knowing how to comb hair is not a requirement of being a certified nursing assistant. She looked sweet and angelic, but that was just an illusion.

Angelic is not how she behaved most days. Maybe she had been sweet and angelic many years ago, but not now. It seems as if she had reverted to a mean and bitter shell of her former self. She frequently yells out profanities and insults. She is known to hit anyone who gets within her reach. Hitting you and then laughing. The hitting has no name on it, and it doesn't matter if you are a staff member or another resident. You're going to be hit, and then she's going to hurl profanities at you in English, Latin, Spanish, and a few other languages.

"futue te ipsi......"flocci non faccio....."

This would carry on all day at times. She wouldn't stop until she lost her voice and became hoarse. Or someone wheeled her back to her room. She didn't seem to like people very much. It seemed as though she preferred to stay in her room all day, talking to herself loudly and usually in some other language. It was our job to encourage socialization. Therefore, we would bring her out of the room to watch television or participate in some activity that might be going on. We knew and were cautious and well aware of her high probability of a fall. If we left her unattended for too long, she would try to stand up and get out of her wheelchair. She could not stand, let alone walk, trying any of them always resulted in a fall, which meant more paperwork for me, calls to her doctor, and her family. "I don't have time for all of that today, it's Friday," I said to myself. So our answer to keeping her fall free was to keep her seated at the Nurses' station under somewhat of a close eye. While she sat there, we simply ignored her profanity and stayed clear of her reach. That is if you didn't want to be hit. This worked out most of the time, and when it didn't, we would "redirect" her. Redirecting was just a fancy word for saying that we distracted her or changed the subject. Today appeared to not be much different from any other day. The only thing that was different today is that I had an admission and had a ton of paperwork to do. I sat at the nurses' desk talking to Mary, one of the nursing assistants, who was sitting in a chair nearby doing some of her paperwork. "This has been a long day. I can't wait to go home." I said to Mary. Just then, I heard a giggle. Mary must have heard it too. At the same time, we both looked up. Mrs. Langford giggled again. We both ignored her.

I continued my charting. She con
as though I could feel her eyes st
would look up, she would look a
"nigger," she whispered.
I look up, she looks away.
"nigger," again, she whispered.
I look up; eyes look the other wa
This was the game this second? I kn
doesn't take away from the uglin
She giggled.
I looked up again.
She looked away.
I looked away.
Then I heard her again, "nigger.
I stared at her, she had a silly lit
It's as if she knew she was getti
beginning to. I try to ignore her a
She starts to giggle loudly. I'd ha
"You're going to your room," I
"Mary, could you please take he
mumbles that she has to run to t
taking her. I get up from my sea
"Let's take you to your room,"
me, she was glad. She didn't lik
anyway. It seemed as though sh
to herself for hours. Taking her

"The time is always right to do the right thing."
-ML King, Jr.

Chapter 3

SOMETIMES WE DON'T CARE ENOUGH

Its 745am, time to begin passing my morning medications. I have 40 patients that I have to give medicines to before 10am.

"Good morning Mr. Lance, time for your medication, here you go, I have them all ready for you in the cup and here is your water."

"Take them yourself cause I don't want them," he says to me.

"Mr. Lance, you know that you need your medicine."

"And it don't matter, cause I still don't want them."

"You know that you need them."

" it's up to you," I say to him.

"I don't care.," he says.

"Fine!" I turn around.

I walk out of the room, dropping the medicine into the toilet and flushing as I pass by. I head to my next resident.

"Good morning Mr. Rogers, time for your medication, here you go, I have them all ready for you in the cup and here is some water."

"Nope and close the door on your way out," he says.

"Ok, have a good day," I say as I walk out of the room. Medicine into the toilet.

"Good morning Mrs. Gantt, I have your medicine, here you go, I have them all ready for you in the cup and here is your water."

"I'm only taking 2 of those pills." She says.

"Fine, it's your choice," I say to her.

"my body, my choice," she responds.

I hand her the cup of pills, she picks through them and takes 2, then drinks a small bit of water. I have no idea which pills she took. I leave the room. Pills into the sharps container.

"Good morning Ms. Dunnlap, I have your medicine, here you go."

I have them all ready for you in the cup, and I have some apple juice for you." She takes them all without a complaint.

"Good morning Ms. Willis, I have your medicine for you." Ms. Willis can't speak, so I put the spoon full of crushed medication mixed with applesauce near her mouth, she opens her mouth and eats them. I give her water to wash them down.

Just then, one of the CNAs comes into the room to tell me that I have a phone call. I lock up my cart. Head to the nurses' station to take the phone call. I return 10 minutes later to continue passing my medications.

"Good morning Mr. Golds, I have your medicine."

He can't speak, so I put the pills in his mouth one by one, he swallows them. I give him water. He swallows.

I take a minute to make the notations in my MAR.

"Good morning Aaron, I have your medicine."

I call him by his first name because he doesn't like to be called Mr. White.

He said that it makes him feel old, he is 76 years old. He just stares at me and opens his mouth; I put the pills into his mouth. He lifts his cup of water, smiles, and then swallows the medicine.

"Thank you, Aaron, have a nice day." I walk out of the room.

"You too, nurse," he says as I close his door.

"Good morning Mr. Ramos, I have your medicine. "

"Did you bring all of this rain?"

I laugh, "No, I didn't. How are you today?"

"I'm fine," he says. I hand him his medication.

"Thanks so much, and have a great day!" I tell him as I turn to leave.

"Have a good day, nurse." He says.

"Thanks, you too." I leave his room.

"Good morning, Mr. Jewels, just letting you know that I'll be bringing your medication in shortly."

"Well, before I take any medication, make sure you have cranberry juice, or I'm not taking any of it."

I look at him. "Mr. Jewels we are out of cranberry juice, I think we have apple juice."

"Well, if you want me to take them pills with apple juice, it better be ice cold, or I'm not taking them ."

I go to the cart and start to "pull" his pills. I Grab the apple juice.

Aggrenox 25
Allopurinol 100mg
Amantadine 100mg
Clonazepam 0.5mg
Colace 250mg
Fish oil 1000mg
Lasix 40mg
Gabapentin 100mg
Generelac 30ml
Klor-con 10 meq
Lisinopril 20mg
Olanzapine 5mg
Oyster shell calcium 500mg with D
Ribavirin 200mg
Vitamin C
I return to his room.

The apple juice is room temperature.

"Mr. Jewels, it's not ice-cold, but it's cool."

"Well, I suggest you go and get some that is cold, or I'm not taking them pills."

I walk out of the room and down the hall to get some cold juice. I return. I place the cold can on his table. He feels it and decides it's cold enough to take with the pills. He looks over the pills and decides to take them.

"Thank you, Mr. Ramos, Have a nice day, sir."

"Next time, I'm not taking them pills if you don't have cranberry juice. I don't like apple juice."

I keep walking.

"ok," I mumble.

"Good morning Mr. Drickery."

"I don't want it," he says.

I immediately turn around and leave his room. Not arguing with him today.

"Have a nice day," I tell him.

No medicine for him this morning.

"Good morning Josephina."

She Immediately starts screaming and kicking at me.

Not today.

I turn around and walk back out of her room.

I hear an overhead page for me.

Another phone call.

"Shit," as I walk to the nurses' station.

I answer the call. Ten minutes with a family member with ten complaints.

I head back to passing my medicine.

"Good m….." I don't fully get the words out of my mouth.

"I don't want it." I turn around and walk back out of the room, "Have a nice day."

"Good morning, Mr. Wade, Mr. Brower."

Mr. Wade doesn't talk, he is one of our total care patients. So is Mr. Brower.

I go to my cart and get Mr. Wade's medicine. I crush all of his medication and put it in applesauce. I grab a cup of water and a straw. I sit down next to him, and I start to give him his medicine. First, a spoonful of medicine, then a sip of water….

"*Oh shit*!" I think as soon as I give him the water.

He starts coughing and spitting it all over me. I FORGOT! He gets thickened liquids. I sit there for about a minute, talking to him and watching him.

Eventually, he calms down, and everything seems to clear.

NO ASPIRATING ON THIS SHIFT. At least I hoped not.

I sit and give him his medicine with thickened water. I'm in this room for an extra 15 minutes because I was rushing and not paying attention. "Okay, Mr. Wade, have a nice day." Of course, he doesn't say anything. I turn and walk out of the room and to my cart to get medicine for Mr. Brower. I return.

"Okay, Mr. Brower, here we go." He stares at me.

"Open your mouth nice and wide." He stares at me.

When I put the spoon near his mouth, he opens. But as soon as he detects the medicine, he quickly closes his mouth and purses his lips!!

He won't open his mouth for medicine.

He loves applesauce. I have to trick him. When his mouth is wide open is when I have to get the medicine in.

It's a game on my part. I've mastered it with him. I call it my two-spoon molly. I have one spoon of plain applesauce and the other with medicine. Kind of, as if when you give a baby peaches and peas…I give him two spoons of applesauce quickly; the third is medicine. I shovel it in.

He smirks. I smile. He swallows. I give him water.

More trickery, spoonful of applesauce, spoonful of medicine, spoonful of applesauce, spoonful of applesauce, spoonful of medicine, finally last spoonful of medicine. All done. "Have a nice day, Mr. Brower." I walk out of the room.

"Good morning Mr. Rogers."

"Good morning nurse, how are you?" he says.

"I'm fine, you taking medicine today?" I ask.

"Oooooh, I might, I might not." He laughs as he talks

"Please don't give me a hard time today." I laugh.

"If I didn't give you a hard time, who would?" I laugh.

"Trust me; I'm going to have a hard time with or without your help." He then takes his medicine. I start to walk out of the room.

"Have a nice day, sir!"

I finally have them all.

"Have a nice day," I say as I am walking out of the room.

I'm too busy for this. I think to myself as I flush the pills down the toilet then walk out of the room.

Her call light comes on 10 minutes later.

The CNA tells me that Mrs. Joseph wants to speak to me.

Are you kidding me, I think to myself.

Down the hall and into her room,

"Yes, Mrs. Joseph?"

"I think I will take my medicine now. I guess I do need them."

IRRITATION overload.

"Okay, Ma'am, let me get them."

"Nurse, do I have to go over there?" says the same confused resident.

"No ma'am you don't, just have a seat and relax." She stares at me.

I go back to the MAR glance over it and pull all of the pills again from the medication cart. I try not to have an attitude as I walk back into the room. She has her towel all laid out. I pour the pills onto the towel just as I had done before.

"Now, can you tell me what they all are and what they are for?" I look at her.

"Mrs. Joseph, take your medication!"

"These are the same pills you have been taking for over 2 years, the same pills I brought to you 15 minutes ago."

"I'm not taking anything unless you tell me what each pill is and what they are for."

I look at her, gather the pills, and put them all into the cup. "When you want your medicine put your call light on, and I will bring them back to you. I begin to walk out of the room.

"You're a stupid bitch, and I think you got your license out of a crackerjack box!!" I don't look back at her.

It's after 9:30am, and I'm not even halfway done.

Sometimes we don't care enough.

Sins of Nurses

"Be kind whenever possible. It is always possible."

-Dalai Lama

Chapter 4

BUSINESS AS USUAL

"God, I'm so sick of Mrs. Willis. I wish she would go to sleep, old bitch, I hope I'm not like this when I get old!" said Pam, a CNA caring for Mrs. Willis.

"Its 2am, I'm tired, and I have to be back here tomorrow for another 16hr shift," says Lisa, the other CNA helping to care for Mrs. Willis.

.Mrs. Willis is 78 years old and has been diagnosed with Dementia and Alzheimers. She wanders the halls looking for an exit that will lead her to her house. She is confused most of the time, she thinks that she is going to work or picking up her children from school; she always has somewhere to go. I'm the nurse on duty, I'm sitting in the nurses' station charting, and in layman's terms that means PAPERWORK, it is what we nurses always seem to have to

No need to say much more, I had been down that road before and trust me, it goes nowhere. Complaining about CNAs, especially ones that are well-liked, goes nowhere with management. I could write another book wholly based on the behaviors of CNA's and the lack of control by management.

Both CNAs jumped up from their comfortable positions, pillows, and blankets falling to the floor. They each stood on the sides of Mrs. Willis; each roughly grabbed her by her frail armpits. She probably didn't weigh more than 110lbs. The two CNAs who were caring for her probably had a combined weight of over 400lbs. off she went, against her will, confused and not understanding. I paid them very little attention; I was too obsessed with trying to complete my charting and to go home on time.

I could only speculate as to what Mrs. Willis may have been thinking as she was handled by these two strangers. Maybe even, wondering where her husband might be? The children? Maybe even her parents. She looked dazed as they carted her back to bed. I could hear her yelling.

OMG, I hope she doesn't wake up the other residents.

I looked up and glanced down the hall again, only to see her hitting at the two CNAs. She was no match.

Hell! Most people would not be a match against those two, and to make matters worse, I don't why, but I just didn't trust them. I had worked with these two before and had felt that they might have crossed the line, a few times. I just couldn't prove it. But deep down I kind of knew.

I continued my charting, and then I noticed that it seemed eerily quiet, probably too quiet. I decided to see what might have been going on down the hall with the two CNAs and Mrs.Willis. I got up from my chair and crept down the hall to check things out. I arrived at Mrs. Willis's room, the door was slightly cracked, I could just barely see inside. I listened quietly at the door, "Stay in this goddamned bed and don't get up again!" I heard one angry voice say.

I then heard the sound of what seemed to be someone falling or landing onto a bed.

"OUCH!" I heard a small cry.

"Don't you get up again!"I heard the other angry voice say.

I quietly opened the door so that I could see inside and peer into the room. Standing over her was each CNA. They both stood on each side of her, holding her down by her arms. She was crying.

I knew it, I thought to myself.

I could see that they were leaning down only a few inches from her face.

I quietly knocked and asked, "Is everything ok?

Each looked back at me and seemed to have smiles on their faces.

" Everything is fine, just getting Mrs. Willis back to bed."

I closed the door and quietly walked away. Mrs. Willis didn't get up again that night.

Sins of Nurses

Mrs. Robinson, her mother, has been in our facility for about 2 months. Two very long months.

Mrs. Robinson is 75 years old, she is alert and is able to speak. Her medical diagnoses are severe Dementia, Alzheimers' Disease, Hypertension, AFib, and Adult Failure to Thrive.

She is probably my least favorite resident to give medicine to. This is in part due to her daughters' constant hovering and attempts to tell you how to correctly perform your job WHILE you are trying to take care of her mother.

The other part that makes it challenging to take care of her is her Dementia and Alzheimers. Both affect her ability to think correctly or to do almost anything. There is nothing that she can do without some kind of assistance or total assistance. She won't call for help, nor request to be taken to the toilet, she is usually unaware that she has even soiled herself.

She has to be checked by the CNAs and the Nurse to make sure that her needs are met. This proves to be a problem in most Nursing Homes.

When the CNAs attempt to check her to make sure that she is clean and dry, she usually doesn't understand that they are there to help her. In her mind, these are two strangers taking her clothes off and touching her in a personal way. There is nothing that we can do to help her think any differently. It just seems that once the human mind is gone, it is gone.

Her history is that prior to the two months at our facility, Mrs. Robinson had been living between the homes of her two daughters, who eventually became unable to care for her. She lived with the first daughter for about a month. It proved to be too overwhelming a job for her. She was then packed up and sent to live with her other daughter. After about two months, the second daughter became overwhelmed and unable to care for her mother, as well. She could not cope with the constant job of caring for someone, even her mother 24 hours a day.

Also, Mrs. Robinson doesn't sleep throughout the night.

Since she's been at our facility, we've noted that she is usually awake most of the night, talking, attempting to climb out of bed, yelling, or even singing.

I imagine she did these things while she was home.

Fast forward, her two daughters appear to be smart and are very knowledgeable when it comes to their mother's care. The two daughters pretty much know everything that should be done when it comes to what the nurses and CNAs should be doing for their mother.

Usually, every day, one of them is there for about an hour or so.

Don't get me wrong, we want involved family members. We just want that involvement to cover all areas. Not just the areas that require your management and direction for the nurses and CNAs. Some of you nurses know what I mean regarding being involved.

Back to my morning med pass. I walk into the room. I have her medication already prepared. Crushed in pudding.

"Good morning Mrs. Robinson, how are you?"

"I'm fine dear, did you see hear that lion roaring during the night?"

"No ma'am, I didn't."

"I have your morning medication, are you ready to take it?"

"Mom, the nurse, needs to give you your medicine, go ahead, and open your mouth for her."

"Don't you think a picture is heavy?" says Mrs. Robinson

"Mrs. Robinson, can you take your medicine for me?"

"Sure, I'll take it. Why is the bird-eating that dog? I don't think my car is ready yet."She looks toward the door.

"Mom, open your mouth," the daughter says.

"Maybe you should try raising the head of the bed a bit "

I tune the daughter out.

I raise the head of the bed slightly.

We go through this everyday and every day the result is the same. She doesn't take it.

"I don't believe that lions should have human babies as pets, do you?" Says Mrs. Robinson

"No, Maam, I don't, can I get you to take some of your medicine?"

"yes, of course, I'll take it,"says Mrs.Robinson

"Maybe you should try coming to this side of the bed….." I tune the daughter out.

Her daughter's eyes are fixed on me and the cup of crushed pills in the pudding. She seems to be becoming increasingly annoyed with this daily process of trying to get her mother to take medication.

I walk around to the other side of the bed, and I again put the spoon near her mouth.

Mrs. Robinson opens her mouth and then closes her mouth. Turns her head, and starts rambling about yarn and mice.

"you know that my mother needs her medicine!" her daughter says in an annoyed voice.

"Yes, Ma'am, I do."

"You also know that we do this every day." I remind her.

I've been in this room for over ten minutes.

She still won't open her mouth to take the medicine.

The daughter continues to stare at me. Not saying a word.

I ask the daughter if she wouldn't mind trying to get her mother to take the medicine. She looks at me as if I have insulted her.

"Isn't that YOUR job to give her medicine? Why are you asking me to do your job?"

I became flushed at her response.

"I just thought that she might take it from you," I say.

In my mind, I'm thinking,

because clearly, I'm incompetent and you can do better.

She continues to stare at me very intensely. Not saying a word to me, the clock is still ticking. I've been here for almost 20 minutes, and as usual, Mrs. Robinson will not take her medicine.

One more attempt and I'm out of here.

I ask her again, trying not to sound impatient.

"Mrs. Robinson, can you please open your mouth for me?" She looks at me with a big smile and says, "Yes, honey, I can, why do you want me to open my mouth?"

I explain to her that I have medicine to give her and that it is good for her.

"Ok," she says.

She opens her mouth. I put some of the medicine on the spoon, and I place it to her mouth.

She opens her mouth and takes it.

She holds the medicine in her mouth, not swallowing.

Someone save me pleaseeeeee

"Mrs. Robinson, could you please swallow the medicine in your mouth?"

She looks at me with a blank stare, and then she looks away. It's still in her mouth. I look at her daughter for help.

"MOM, swallow the medicine, please ...Mom open your mouth."

She doesn't. She simply stares at us both. The pudding and medication mixture is slowly oozing from the corner of her pursed lips.

"Just let me have it." The daughter says.

The hand the daughter the spoon and cup of medicine.

"Mom, open your mouth!"

Mrs. Robinson smiles.

The daughter tries to shovel a spoonful of medicine in her mouth.

Mrs. Robinson turns her head with a smile.

The daughter is turning red with frustration.

I'm simply standing there watching the whole thing.

"MOM,!" she yells

"Yes, dear?" medicine running out of her mouth.

"Those spoons have to be put into the car before that mouse gets them." Mrs. Robinson says.

If I weren't getting so behind, I would have laughed.

"Yes, Maam."

I had my" best actress nominated as a 'serious' nurse" face on.

"Now what?" the daughter asks in a very frustrated voice.

Sins of Nurses

"Roses, rainbows, kittens, and shit!"

-R.L Green

Chapter 6

THIS DAY

"Here we go today with Nurse Green and her bullshit!" I hear one of the nursing assistants say loud enough for me to hear as they walk outside for their break. I tune them out.

"Nurse, Mrs. Brown says she needs a pain pill, "says another nursing assistant.

"Ok, tell her to give me a few minutes, and I'll be right there."

At the nurses' station, Mr. Crohm is yelling!

"Help help help! Someone help me, help help help!"

I look to his direction. He is sitting in the common area, along with several other residents.

Mr. Morgan, who can barely stand, let alone walk, is standing and attempting to walk.

"Mr. Morgan, have a seat, please, sit down in your wheelchair!" I yell to him. He looks up at me and sits.

My hands are full. I'm attempting to spike and hang my IV Vancomycin for another resident. In the distance and somewhere down the hall I hear

|" ma'am ma'am ma'am ma'am ma'am ma'am can you hear me? Ma'am ma'am?" Mr. Martin, again.

I'm trying to concentrate on hanging this antibiotic. I look around the common area to see my residents in varying stages of positioning and stress.

Mr. Glenn is sliding out of his wheelchair.

"Mr. Glenn, sit up straight please and stop sliding," I exclaim.

He looks at me and haphazardly pulls himself back into his wheelchair. I catch Mrs. Bloward out of the corner of my eye.

"Mrs. Bloward, sit down, please. Mrs. Bloward, you're going to fall!"

"Nurse, can you get me a towel?' says a resident.

"Give me a minute." I quickly go to the linen cart and grab her a towel.

"Here you go."

"You didn't wet it." She says

I look around for a CNA, they are still hanging around outside.

"Help helpppp helppppp helpppppp helppppppp!"

I go into the nearest room, wet the towel, and bring it back to her.

"It's warm! I wanted it cold." She says.

I leave her with the towel and walk away.

Back to the Nurses station to finish priming my IV tubing.

I look up, Mrs. Glenn again.

I throw everything on the counter and run to her.

No falls today.

I pull her up by the seat of her pants and back into the chair.

Then back to my IV, priming my tubing, no air bubbles.

"Nurse Green I need you, Ms. Jones is on the floor."

"Ma'am ma'am ma'am ma'am maammmmmmm!"

The yelling continues.

"Help helppppp helppppp helpppppp helppppppp!"

"SHUT UP!" another resident yells.

I'm heading down the hall to Ms. Jones' room.

"I heard her yelling and found her sitting here." says the CNA.

"Could you please grab her vitals for me?"

I perform a quick assessment; nothing appears broken. She's fine.

As I walk out of the room and back to the nurses' station, the nursing assistant from earlier approaches me again.

"Nurse, Mrs. Brown is still waiting for her pain pill."

Let her know that I'm making my way to her shortly, please.

I hear a g-tube pump alarming from one of the rooms.

"ma'am ma'am ma'am maaaaam!" the yelling continues.

At that moment, Mrs. Brown rolls up to me in her motorized wheelchair. She is staring me down with intensity and anger.

"I know the CNA told you that I needed my oxycontin!"

Before I can say anything, she says, "I don't know how you got a license to become a nurse, but they need to take it back from you!"

I force a smile, "Let me get it now."

I hear her mumble, "bitch!"

I turn to her, "Did you say something?"

She simply glares at me. I turn and head toward the med cart to get her oxycontin and ALL of her other medicine.

...*BITCH*....I mumble to myself.

"I'll be waiting in my room." She turns and rolls away.

"Where do I go?" a resident says.

'Your room is down the hall, Charlie."

Charlie turns to head down the hall to his room. He makes it about halfway and returns to me.

"Where should I go?"

"Charlie, your room is down the hall, and to the left, you should head that way; your name is on the door."

"ok," he says. He begins to walk toward his room.

The g-tube pump is still beeping.

Mrs. Brown is still waiting and staring at me from the door of her room.

Another resident, Mrs. Allen, is unfastening her seat belt/safety belt so that she can stand. The belt looks like a regular seat, but it's purpose is to act as a deterrent to her standing. A shrieking alarm rings when the belt is unfastened. She is confused, but she knows how to unfasten this belt. The alarm shrieks. If she is unsupervised and allowed to stand, she will definitely fall.

"Mrs. Allen!" I run to her and fasten the seat belt.

"Just have a seat over there, ma'am," I tell another confused and wandering resident as she wanders away.

I hurry to Mrs. Brown to give her medicine. She snatches the pills and the cup of water from me. She takes all of the medicine and then wheels away, not saying a word.

"*youre welcome.*" She doesn't look back.

"Help helppppp helpppp helpppppp!" the yelling continues.

"Good morning," says the Director of Nursing with a big smile on her face as she heads inside her office.

Her nose is in the air; she doesn't see or hear anything.

"Mrs.Bloward! SIT DOWN!"I yell.

The Director of Nursing steps out of her office and smiles her biggest brightest smile.

"Don't forget your Medicare charting."

"Any chance you can work dayshift tomorrow?"

Says the staffing coordinator as she walks by.

"No, sorry, I can't."

No CNAs insight, still on breaks, together.

The DON sees nothing that concerns her, she's waiting for my acknowledgment regarding the medicare charting.

"ok," I answer.

The DON returns to her office, the chaos continues.

I run to silence the beeping g-tube pump.

Its empty, *thanks night shift.*

The wheelchair safety belt for Mr. Allen is alarming.

Have you ever noticed how management usually doesn't have much to say to you, barely even a smile until they want something like, "can you work an extra shift?"

I'm over that fake niceness. When I want to address problems with the cna's, staffing, lack of supplies, inappropriate behaviors, ...they are almost rude. Again, unless it benefits them.

Back into her office, she strolls.

I go to Mr. Allen and gently push him back into a sitting position as I reconnect his safety belt.

"Ma'am ma'am ma'am ma'am ma'am ma'am!"

Think happy thoughts. Six more hours.

"MRS. BLOWARD!!!"

I run to her. I catch her just in time. I glance down the hall. The same nursing assistants are still sitting outside. I haven't seen another one.

"Today is going to be a good day; today is going to be a good day."

The common area smells heavily of urine.

"Where should I go?" Charlie again.

"Sir, just have a seat in that chair," I tell him again.

Mr. Glenn slides out of his wheelchair and onto the floor. I go over and help him back into the wheelchair. He reeks of urine, and his pants are heavily soiled.

His CNA casually walks by.

"Mr. Glenn needs to be changed," I say to her.

She rolls her eyes at me. "I hope you're not going to start today Nurse Green!"

I ignore her.

Don't start expecting you to do your job today, I know.

"Help help help help somebody help me!"

"Mr. Martin, what do you need help with? Mr. Martin!"

He stares at me. He continues to yell.

The Administrator walks by with all of her papers. Smiling.

"Good morning Mrs. Bloward."She says.

Mrs. Bloward is attempting to stand.

I yell, "SIT DOWN, MRS. BLOWARD!"

The Administrator keeps walking. She doesn't see anything, and since her nose is so far into the air, she doesn't smell the urine.

"ma'am ma'am ma'am ma'am ma'am ma'am ma'am!"

What time is it? I look at the clock. It's 8:30am I've been here since 6:30am, and I haven't gotten a thing accomplished

No one is around. One incident report to do. I haven't even started my med pass. The kitchen staff is bringing out the breakfast trays. Their very late today. They leave them in the hall. I gather all of my supplies and walk down the hall to Mr. Golden's room, where I'm going to hang his IV antibiotics. I look around the room. It's dirty, stains on the floor and walls, a fly is sitting on his knee, the strong odor of urine is present. He's just lying there. Physically there, but not there.

"Good morning Mr. Golden, I'm going to be giving you an antibiotic through that port in your arm."

His head turns toward me. He looks at me. His face and skin look dirty. His lips are cracked and dry. He's lying crookedly in the bed. I look into his eyes with despair. He looks back with despair.

How did I get here?

What are we doing?

How did he get here?

I go back to hanging my IV antibiotics.

Mr. Arris, his roommate, is mumbling something as he flops into his wheelchair. He looks at me and says something. I can't understand him. He has a very heavy Italian accent. Mr. Arris is psychotic and needs to be heavily medicated most of the time. For the safety of everyone. He wheels himself out of the room, mumbling to himself. I continue to hang my IV antibiotic. Mr. Golden still has his eyes glued on me, not saying a word. I smile at him. He stares. He has a PICC line. I flush the blue port and connect the tubing. I set the pump, IV is primed and running. I can still hear the yelling from the hall. I walk to my med cart.

"Nurse could you get me some water, I'm thirsty."

I barely look her way, I smile.

"Sure"

I take her cup, down the hall to the other end of the building, to get a cup of ice and water. I feel numb. I bring the ice water back to her.

"Thank you, Nurse."

"You're welcome."

Mr. Arris is on my heels yelling. "Give me my medicine."

Back to the cart, pulling the medications for Mr. Arris.

Multivitamin with minerals

Amantadine 100mg

Keppra 500mg

Depakote 500mg

Geodon 60mg

Lactulose 30ml

Vitamin C 250mg

Pepcid 20mg

Chlordiazepoxide 25mg

Tramadol 50mg

Miralax

Colace

Norvasc 10mg

I hand the small cup filled with pills to him. He swallows all of the pills in one mouthful with a sip of the miralaxed water.

"Where's my cough syrup?"

I pour him cough syrup and hand the small cup to him, I don't think he even has an order for cough syrup any longer.

Geri-tussin 20cc

Did you give me my pain pill?

"Yes, I did."

He wheels away in his wheelchair.

"Maam ma'am ma'am, can anyone hear me?

Everyone keeps walking, no one acknowledges him.

Two nursing assistants are passing out breakfast trays. They roll their eyes at me, implying that I shouldn't ask them to do anything else.

I head to my medication cart to start my med pass. It's almost 9 am.

This day is no different from any other day.

Sins of Nurses

Choose a job you love, and you will never have to work a day in your life."   - Confucius

Chapter 7

G-TUBES AND CONTRACTURES

One of the hardest things to do is to give medication to a patient who is confused, contracted and has a g-tube. Nothing too special about it from a mental perspective. It's the physical acrobatics that you have to master. I can think of countless stories and countless times that I've had to give medicine to patients like this. Anyway, it's 8am, and I'm giving my 9am medications. I have 25 patients. 5 have tubes of some kind, 5 are confused and require extensive care and assistance, 10 are alert and oriented X 3 as we say, requiring minimal care and the last 5 are somewhere between alert and sound, *and alert and well, just alert.* Either way, they all need their medication, and I have 2 hours to give it. It's 8am, and I push my cart down the hall to the first room. I don't know if I want to get my day started with this particular resident, Mrs. Royce. I think to myself, "Should I save the worst for last or should I do the worst first and get it over with?" Forget it, I'll start here. Mrs. Royce is mean; she pinches, hits, spits, yells, and screams. She is a large woman who has a g-tube, is bedbound and has contractures to her arms and legs. Her body has grown to form a fetal position. I'm waiting outside of her door for the CNA who has this room assignment to help me; starting by myself is not an option. Stacey arrives to help. We put on gloves, Stacey puts on a gown. This is going to be 15 minutes, and I'm done, I hope. We enter the room, and as soon as she sees us, she begins to yell AND scream, flailing contracted arms and legs in protest. We haven't even touched her.

"Jeesh! We haven't even gotten started," says Stacey.

We close the door and pull her privacy curtain. Stacey goes to her right, I go to the left. We let the head of the bed up a bit more. She immediately starts with her usual high-pitched screaming. If a visitor or family member were walking anywhere near the room, they might think that we were doing something harmful to her. In her mind, I guess we were. I have too much to do today for Mrs. Royce. I think I'll just start with her blood pressure. I'm trying to put the blood pressure cuff on her arm. She is fighting me as much as she can. I can't get the cuff on her arm. I can't even get it on her wrist.

It's not going to happen. I give up.

"Forget it, Stacey" We both shake our heads. Next Task.

"Ok, Mrs. Royce, I'm going to start your feeding now."

Stacey begins to pull and turn her so that I can try to give her the medication and nutritional supplement through her g-tube. The thing is, I have to check her g-tube for placement first.

It would be nice if I could even get to her g-tube.

She is attempting to bite and spit at the two of us, and she won't stop flailing about. Stacey is trying to hold her still. She is practically in bed with her. I've got my stethoscope out, and I'm trying to check the placement, I'm attempting to listen to the air that I'm ATTEMPTING to put into her stomach.

This is not working.

"I think that we are going to need another person to help with her today. " says Stacey.

"Ok, let's just stop. "I say.

Stacey goes to find another CNA.

I go to the door and peer out, hoping someone will happen by. No luck. The usual, not a CNA in sight. I turn on her call light.

Stacey returns, "everyone is busy."

It's back to Stacey and myself.

Stacey is holding her for me.

I decide to skip the whole process of checking and making sure that the tube is in place with my stethoscope. I choose to simply connect the syringe and aspirate for any stomach contents, looks like just a couple of cc's.

CLOSE ENOUGH!! *I need to get this over with*!

Stacey is practically in the bed sitting on top of her, holding her arms and legs. I barely have room to work. I flush her tube with some water. Then I draw up some of the medication into the piston syringe. I manage to get some of the medicine into her stomach; she is still squirming and flailing. She somehow grabs me by the arm and proceeds to hold on for dear life. Her nails are digging into my arm, and I'm practically in the bed with her.

"goddamit!!" mumble to myself.

I manage to wrestle away from her, *barely*. I look at my arm, no blood. Just some scratches that are starting to turn red and sting.

"Dammit, this is going to be paperwork."

Let me get this done."

I manage to give her the balance of her medication. I then begin trying to give her the supplement through the tube. It's a bolus feeding. Which means it's a balancing act.

The way that she is fighting us, it's a miracle I am able to get anything down her tube.

There is no easy way to manage a patient like this.

I digress.

Anyway, I have two large cups. One is a large cup of water. The other a large cup of which I've poured the contents of one of my cans.

I'm the juggling nurse at this point.

I manage to get the first can into the tube and into her stomach. She seems to have calmed down a bit; never mind I spoke too soon.

She is starting to yell, spit, and scratch at us. I stay out of the line of her spitfire as best as I can. I was too lazy to put on a gown to protect myself, I'm regretting that decision. I start with the second can, slowly pouring, pouring....She suddenly gets a burst of extra energy. Her arms flail, and her body lifts. Stacey loses her hold, I let go of the tube, the syringe, the cup of water. ...and at that moment....for some odd reason I hear the voice from bikini bottom go through my head... I stumble backward/forward; everything flies! Stomach contents, water, cup, the milky supplement, and me. Everywhere! All over the bed, the floor, the wall, her, Stacey, and me.

"Motherfucking, are you kidding me?" Stacey yells. Although she has a gown on to offer some protection, it doesn't do the trick. She has a small amount of the milky supplement on her face and hands. Me, on the other hand, I'm covered.....

"motherfuck !!!" I curse loudly.

We let go of Mrs. Royce. I look down at myself. I want to cry.

How can my day be starting like this?

"I'll be right back," Stacey mumbles as she leaves the room to get towels and clean linen. I'm looking at Mrs. Royce, covered in water and supplement, she's looking at me. She's no longer fighting and spitting, I guess she's in shock also. I look at the clock. Typically I might have left the room and left Stacey to any small mess. But not today. I was responsible for this one, and it was a big one.

"No, no, nooo! " I can't be starting my shift off this way.

Stacey returns, and we start the cleanup, we look at each other and shake our heads. I don't bother trying to give another can of the supplement. I'm way behind with giving my medications. I help Stacey do most of the cleanup and the linen changing. I feel gross. I'm sticky, and now I'm hot. Stacey is cursing the whole time. We get everything cleaned up. It's done, finally. Now to change my clothes. I walk out of the room and into the hall. I head to my car for my spare uniform. I'm walking down the hall, stained and sticky. The other nurse that I'm working with is laughing, the other CNAs are laughing. NOW there are people around.

"What happened?" they're laughing at the same time.

I ignore them.

Good thing I have another uniform in my car.

I grab the uniform from my car and into the bathroom I go. I quickly wash/wipe and dry off as best as I can. I put on my wrinkled clean uniform and head back to the room of Mrs. Royce debating. I really should give her another can of her supplement.

I look at her, she starts to yell.

I turn around and walk away. I decide not to do anything else with her.

I return to my med cart, its 8:15am. One patient down, 24 to go.

Sins of Nurses

“Two things are infinite: the universe and human stupidity; and I’m not sure about the universe.”

-Albert Einstein

Chapter 8

THE RAISED BED

I was sitting at the nurses when they brought him in, pushing him in a wheelchair. Two police officers, an EMS team, and what looked to be a social worker accompanied him. He was cursing up a storm.

"You can't do this!"

"You stupid motherfuckers!"

"I know my rights!"

"My daughter doesn't have the authority to do this!"

Here we go, I thought to myself

Apparently, he was being placed into the nursing home based on a court order which declared him incompetent, his daughter, who was downstairs in the building,, signing all of the paperwork. He was found to be living in filthy, uninhabitable conditions similar to hoarding. He appeared to be mentally unstable, had bedsores, and wasn't able to take care of himself. This was to be my admission.

Thanks, Joan, in Admissions!

I follow the EMS team down to his room. I grab a CNA along the way, ...a male. I knew that I would need a male CNA to help me with him once the police officers left.

We arrive at his room.

The social worker tries to reason with him. He continues to yell profanity at her.

She throws her hands up and leaves to talk to his daughter. It remains just him, the male CNA, and me.

I start to introduce myself. He begins cursing me and tells me that he wasn't going to be staying here for long. I try to get a medical history on him. He won't cooperate at all. I'm not sure what I am working with. He could have high blood pressure, diabetes, heart problems, who knew. The only thing that we did know is that he had bedsores and leg wounds. He had old and dried bandages on his legs; they looked like they've been there for some time. We leave him in the room in the wheelchair, hoping that he will adjust to the idea that he's stuck with us, and we're stuck with him. I return a short time later, and I ask him if he's hungry.

"get out!" He yells.

I return an hour later. He should be calm by now.

"Sir, are you hungry? Can I get you something to eat?"

"sure," he says as if I continue to annoy him.

I order him a food tray with a variety of things for him to eat and drink, and I take it to his room. I place it in front of him, and then I leave.

I check back 30 minutes later.

Looks like he's eaten everything and what he hasn't eaten, he's stashed in a backpack lying next to his bed.

He seems a bit more agreeable this time.

"Mr. Johnson, I really need to look at your legs so that we can take care of them. You think that you could just show me how you take care of your wounds at home?"

To my surprise, he agrees. I go to grab supplies, but I change my mind and decide to bring the whole cart.

I'm not sure what supplies I'm going to need.

I arrive at the room, and he's ripping off bandages and exposing yellow-green (pus-like), blood, slimy, foul, and odorous wounds. I want to vomit from the smell.

Actually, it's not the worst that I've ever seen, so no point in vomiting.

He's wiping the wounds and the drainage with toilet tissue that is sticking to the wounds. I'm horrified. I offer to help, but he refuses. I hand him some bandages. He sloppily wraps his right leg. I watch as he does the same to his left leg.

He's rambling on the whole time about a dog and a cat and then a rat. I couldn't follow his story.

"*why meeeeee,*" I shake my head.

He then pulls down his shorts, turns on his side, and removes a big wad of tissue from his butt area.

(At least I think its tissue)

It's soaked with the same foul-smelling drainage as his legs. He simply folds up what looks like a half roll of tissue and then stuffs it.

"Mr. Johnson, let me help you!"

"Don't touch me. I can do this. !"

As best I can, I've taken a few notes regarding the drainage and my guess on the size of the wounds that I've seen. When he finishes, he pulls a handkerchief from his pocket, spits on his hands, and wipes his hands. He looks closer. He then spits on one of his fingers and wipes it clean.

I smile and thank him.

I leave his room and call the doctor. I explain the situation and my findings. He gives me orders, including orders to forcibly (if necessary) change his dressings.

(It's not done as much nowadays, but it happens)

It meant that we were going to use whatever means needed to assess the wound on his butt and then change the dressings DAILY.

Thank God, my shift is almost over, this is going to be an evening and night shift problem, and I won't be here for the drama of it all. When I return the next day, the night nurse gives me the details on how it took three CNA's to hold him down while the nurse assessed and measured all of his wounds. She says he hit, cursed, spit on everyone, and then called the police.

"What?" I exclaim.

She laughs and says that he called the police from his cell phone and that they had come out, did a report, and left.

"OMG!!!" I exclaimed.

So this was our introduction to Mr. Johnson and the start of our hate-hate relationship.

Immediately, Mr. Johnson became the hoarder that he had been at home. His daughter would bring him food; it would pile in the room. He wouldn't take baths or showers. Once a week, by force, we took him to the shower, and forcibly gave him one. The only thing he had learned to cooperate with us on.... was his dressing changes, and he would let us do those daily. As the days passed, HE decided that it was best to keep his bed elevated at its highest height while he was in it. He did this whenever he could. This posed a safety hazard for us. We first began by asking him nicely to lower his bed. He hurled profanities and still refused. We grew tired of asking him, so we took matters into our own hands. We decided to help him out and do it for him. He would cuss, fight, and complain. Whenever we passed his room and noticed that his bed was elevated at its maximum height, we would lower it. If he fell from the bed at its maximum height, he would surely break something. We were over it either way. Someone got an idea, and we couldn't wait to test it. He raised the bed, and we lowered the bed. We then went one step further by disconnecting the power controller and placing it on the other side of the room where he couldn't get to it. We came back later and checked on him. He had raised the bed again.

"Son of a bitch!!"

I attempted to retrieve the controller to lower the bed. He's hidden it. I stare at him,

"Give me that controller, where is it?"

"I'm not giving you a goddam thing, get the hell outta here!"

I looked around his room and didn't see it anywhere. I know that he will probably hit me with something if I get too close, so I go to get help. I returned to his room with two nursing assistants, and we searched for the controller. It was under his pillow. We take it, lower the bed, and carry the controller back to the nurses' station. This went well for a few days. He was pissed during this time. He then started coming out of the room and sitting at the nurses' station, yelling and cursing at anyone who passed by him. It didn't matter if it were another resident or staff member. One day he got so upset with us for not giving him the bed controller that he called the police again! They came out. Another report and then they left. A few days later, I went by his room, and to my shock, there he sat with the bed elevated.

What the hell? Here we go again!

I got to the Nurses station, and there sat the bed controller.

What the heck!

How did he get his bed up without the controller?

I go for back up!

We search the room and find a bed controller.

We lower the bed.

We then figured out that he had gone into one of the empty rooms and had figured out that the bed controllers were pretty universal.

All of the nurses complained to the unit manager about him. I told one of the other nurses that I was so tired of complaining to the unit manager with nothing being done. The days go by, and if we have lowered the bed he gets out of the bed and into his wheelchair, stealing the bed remotes out of any resident room

It was irritating.

I was working one evening and noticed that his bed was elevated at its maximum height again.

"Shit," he's stolen another remote from someone.

I told the nurse that I was working with all about it.

She thought it was funny; she couldn't stop laughing. Eventually, I started laughing as we shook our heads. I waited for him to fall asleep. I crept into the room and grabbed the remote. This time I left the bed elevated at its maximum height. He must have awakened, searched for the remote, couldn't find it, and realized that one of us had probably taken it while he was sleeping. He yelled for us to let his bed down. We all ignored him. A short time later, we heard a horrible "thud" sound and the crashing of things hitting the floor. We ran to his room to see him lying on the floor. His leg appeared turned at a weird angle.

"Oh shit!" We didn't move him.

I placed a pillow under his head while the CNA grabbed the equipment to check his vital signs. I knew that he was going to need to be sent to the hospital. I left him with the CNA telling her that I was going to start his paperwork to send him to the hospital. When I left, he was moaning in pain, yelling, and hurling profanities. I looked down the hall, no one was headed my way yet. I looked back and noticed the bed. I ran to the room across the hall, grabbed the remote, attached it to his bed, and lowered it. The CNA returned and started taking his vital signs. I told her that I would be back in a few

"I'm going to make sure his paperwork is ready."

The other nurse had begun the process of calling the doctor for orders to send him to the hospital and calling for an ambulance. I started working on the transfer paperwork to send him to the hospital. I took his paperwork back to the room and was looking it over when the EMS team arrived to transport him to the hospital. They put him on a stretcher, and began to wheel him down the hall; all that you could hear him say was

"That fucking bitch left my bed up, and I fell out."

"They stole my remote!!"

The EMS person looked at me. I didn't comment, I gave him the paperwork.

After they left, I sat down to write up the incident report as to what had happened. I was very thorough and detailed in my account as to what may have happened. No one was in the room with him, so we aren't sure what happened. We do know that it was bound to happen with him raising that bed up all the time.

When we called to check on him, they said that his leg was broken and that he would remain in the hospital for surgery to repair it.

****Sins of Nurses****

"If you tell the truth, you don't have to remember anything."

-Mark Twain

Chapter 9

THIEF

In almost every career field, there is abuse, abuse of some kind, forging documents, paperwork, time-lines, time clocks, payroll, favoritism, harassment, stealing.......... STEALING!! Some people will take something/anything from where they work. It could be an ink pen or two, food from the restaurant where they are employed, a box of highlighters, material from a construction site, a coworkers lunch, packets of folders .... copy paper. It's just a fact of the times that we live in. Some people have a false sense of entitlement. Some take things simply because the opportunity presents itself, and they can. Others feel that they deserve something from their employers who underpay them. Still, others steal out of necessity to get by.

Nursing is no different. I was a divorced woman with three children. I didn't make a whole lot of money. I grew up on the south side of Chicago. Starting around September, at the start of the school year, I would always work for a temporary staffing agency.

Usually, I tried for a pediatric clinic. I would pick up as many shifts as often as I could. *Why?* Pediatric clinics had lots of pharmaceutical samples of everything from Tylenol, Motrin, Robitussin, and even nasal spray. They stocked the latest cold medicines, newest medication for ear infections, antibiotics, eye infections, you name it...

I had a system when I worked.

I would always ask the nurse whom I was working with if it would be ok to take a few samples from the cabinets. The answer was usually yes. The clinics didn't usually mind. It didn't matter if they did mind.

I would steal them if I had to.

I'd ask for Tylenol samples, saying that one of my children had a fever or something, and then I'd take a few samples of anything else that I thought I might need. A few weeks of doing this, and I almost always had enough to last me through the winter months of Chicago. I'm not proud of this, but I did what I had to do. I didn't have time to take off from work for sick kids, I couldn't afford the loss to my income. I didn't have insurance for three children. Many nurses without insurance treat their children at home, rather than run to emergency rooms or wait for expensive pediatric appointments. I've talked to lots of nurses in writing this book and have taken many notes. I have compared many of the things that many of us have done. There are some bad things that I have done and would do again if I had to. But then there are some things that I view as really bad and would never do as a nurse. Stealing from a resident is one of them. This brings me to the point of my story.

I had a good friend who was a nurse. She was an outstanding nurse, but she regularly made terrible decisions in men. She was always in some form of an abusive relationship. Whomever, the boyfriend, was; was always either taking her money or hitting her. I know that many of us have had financial difficulties at some point in our lives. But Celia had quite a few may be more than most. Depending on whom you asked.

We had been friends for years, and I thought that I knew her. But I soon realized that I really didn't. I knew that she was a thief.

How did I know? You ask.

Well, she was always stealing something; small things, but always something. I thought that it was funny for a while. She stole everything; rolls of tissue from the bathroom, trash bags, paper towels, food from the kitchen, anything that could be used in her home she stole it. She was that employee who stole other peoples' lunch out the fridge. One day as she stuffed one of her big bags with stolen items, I jokingly said to her, “at least you don’t steal from the patients.”

She gave me a funny look.

“Nooo, please tell me you don’t steal from the patients.”

She simply replied,

"You know I’m a thief," She then burst into laughter.

I thought to myself, *stealing supplies and drinks was one thing, but taking from people was another.*

I was shocked.

Nevertheless, I guess I shouldn’t have been.

She went on to tell me that she had a couple of stories for my book and that she will call me to tell me about them later.

“I can’t wait to hear all about it.”

She called me at home that night. I grabbed a glass of wine, knowing this was going to be interesting. She started by saying,

“So, you know that I quit my part-time job last week?”

I remembered she called me last week pretty upset and said that she had quit her job. A temporary position on a private duty case that she had been working for the past few months. Last week she hadn’t told me why she had quit. She had only said that she didn’t want to talk about it. I left it alone, not wanting to press the issue. Tonight she tells me that she had not quit but that she had been fired. She said that she had been working a private duty case taking care of an elderly woman in her home. That one evening, her patient had asked her to read a book. She agreed and grabbed a book. When she opened, the page there was a $100 bill between the pages.

She said that she asked herself.

Should I leave it or keep it, no one will notice it missing.

She said she decided to keep it and that once her patient had gone to sleep, she began to go through a few more books and found another $100 bill. She said that from that moment, she realized the kind of person she was caring for, and from that point, every time she worked, and the woman went to sleep, she searched through her things and would find $100s of dollars.

This went on for weeks.

Fast forward. At the end of her shift, the last time that she had worked, the patients' son and his wife asked to speak to her.

They sat her down. The son began by saying how great a Nurse that she was with his mother, BUT that he knew that she had been stealing from her. That he knew that there had been monies hidden by his mother in her earlier years and that it was no secret to their family. He said that he knew that there was probably money all over the house and that the family had decided to leave the money in place. He went on to say that, by chance, he had noticed that money from a particular book was gone. He stated that he checked a few other places and noticed that the money was gone from those places as well.

That they had noticed that the money had begun to disappear, particularly after she worked her shifts. She attempted to protest, but the son stopped her and asked her not to. He then said that he would not report her to her agency and that she did not have to worry about paying the money back. They simply asked that she not return to his mother's home.

She said that she sat quietly and silently, trying to think of something to say.

Nothing came to mind, many things came to mind.

She stood and gathered her things and attempted to leave gracefully.

I listened and was speechless.

"My feeling embarrassed would be an understatement."

she said.

I just kept asking myself how I had not realized that my friend was this type of person. A true thief.

I didn't know what to say to her after hearing this. She then went on to say that she had another thing to confess, and then she seemed to laugh nervously.

"There's more?" I asked.

"I steal from the people at the hospital too, but not the patients, it's their family members."

"What!!!" I exclaimed,

why is she confessing to me? I have my own problems.

I couldn't believe what I was hearing. I listened silently.

She then went on to explain to me how she had done this.

"Okay, so you know how family members come up to visit and sit doing nothing?" I nod at the phone.

"Yeah, okay," I guess.

She said that whenever a family member would come to visit, she would look at their clothes, shoes, purses, suits, all to ascertain as to whether they appeared to have money. The purse, the shoes, the clothes…it all makes a financial statement. She said that if she determined that a family had money, usually the female member, she would tell that family how important exercise was to the resident and encourage them to walk the resident down the halls a few times.

Many hospitals will encourage family members to do this at times.

It wasn't uncommon.

She said that she would then tell the family that they could leave their belongings in the room and that she would close the door. Once the resident and the family members would start down the hall, she would then make a grand production of closing the door.

A false sense of security.

Most people don't realize that rooms can have a connecting door for a resident next door. Even if they notice these doors, they don't connect the two.

Just think about it. When you are visiting someone in the hospital, you don't think much of doors and connecting rooms.

She said that once the patient and the family member were down the hall, she would then go through the connecting door and back into the person's room where she would go through the purse and steal cash.

Eventually, she said, she became brave enough to even a steal one of their credit cards.

She would then sell these cards to credit card thieves.

I was again speechless, I was silent on the phone with her.

"oh my God, you're a fucking low life thief" is what I wanted to say.

I didn't, I was silent.

I had never had a professional person tell me such a thing. She said that the reason that she was telling me this is because she needed to talk to someone. That a family member had accused her of stealing and that she might be fired, she was being investigated by the hospital. Even though she denied the accusations, the family member was adamant that her items had been stolen while at the hospital and that this nurse, my friend, was the only person that could have stolen her credit card and money.

I held the phone. My jaw had dropped.

"Say something." She kept saying.

"I don't know what to say," was my response.

"I'll call you back later." I said as I hung up.

I didn't call her back.

The next day when I arrived for my shift, I saw her for a brief second. We walked toward each other. I was going to ask her how things were going. Just at that moment, she was called to the supervisors' office.

She whispered, "wish me luck," as she got on the elevator.

I remember seeing her later; she was leaving the building with her things. Later that day, she paged me. She had also left a message on my answering machine that night. I didn't answer, and I didn't call her back. When I went in to work the next day people were talking. I felt that they were wondering if I might be a thief as well. No one ever asked me about her, and I never commented about her. I saw her years later when I was pregnant with my son.

She had gained a lot of weight, probably 60-70lbs. I almost didn't recognize her. We chatted for a few; she said that she wasn't doing nursing anymore. That she was now doing real estate.

"oh, that's good," I aid.

I didn't ask her why she had left nursing for real estate. We promised that we would do lunch soon. I never called her, she didn't call me.

Sins of Nurses

"Try to believe what is told to you as truth, even if you don't see it with your own eyes?"

-R.L Green

Chapter 10

THINGS A CNA WILL DO IN A BAD NURSING HOME

1. Take a resident's food tray while they are still eating.
2. Push wheelchairs, yell at residents, feed residents, clean poop all while holding on to their cell phones talking.
3. Six cna's standing at the Nurses' station; a resident approaches with his pants falling down. The pants fall to the floor, he tries to walk away, unsteady, no balance, almost falling; they continue their conversation, no one moves to help. (myself and another Nurse actually witnessed this)
4. Wear inappropriately tight fitted scrubs/uniforms to the point of barely being able to move or bend, but they've clocked in for work.
5. Leave the floor and not tell anyone, run to their children's school, return 2 hours later as if they never left.
6. Sit in the room occupied by two residents, and speak their native language, laughing, and talking. While the residents look on strangely.
7. Sit in a residents' room in their personal recliner and watch tv.
8. Sit in a residents' room and watch Netflix on their phone while call lights are going off.
9. Ask the nurse every day for two Tylenol.

10. Sit at the Nurses' station more than the Nurse.

11. Sit at the Nurses' station and won't move and let the Nurse have a seat.

12. Twerk down the halls.

13. Fight another a Nurse or another CNA

14. Flatten the tires of a Nurse

15. Rarely give residents water even when instructed to do so.

16. Pretend to give residents water

17. Yell at residents

18. Use Profanity toward residents

19. Tell management that the Nurse has something personal against them when the nurse tries to enforce policy and writes him/her up.

20. Arrive at their shift late and immediately go on a break.

21. LIE on a resident

22. LIE on a nurse

23. Threaten a Nurse

24. Eat a residents' personal food

25.Conspire to have a good Nurse fired

26. Shed fake tears when they are caught in a lie

"The opposite of love is not hate, its' indifference."

-Eliezer Wiesel

Chapter 11

DORIS

Doris was 74 years old, with a medical diagnosis of mild dementia, nothing much was wrong with her if you overlooked the fact that she was sneaky and mean as hell. She was a thinly built woman with long white wiry hair. Doris beat up everyone she came in contact with. It didn't matter if it were a nurse, a cna, or even another resident. Doris didn't care.

I don't recall much of her personal background. I believe she was somewhat of a recluse before coming to our facility some years ago. Maybe there was something in her past that had made her this way; sneaky and mean.

Immediately upon being hired, I was warned to beware of Doris and to not turn your back on her. My first thought is that she was not appropriate for this particular floor, an Alzheimer's unit. I've noticed that in these recent years there has been a trend in facilities to make money by any means necessary. AKA Accept as many residents as possible, especially if they were private pay, and I believe that Doris had money from some resource like a trust fund. In that trend to accept any patient, and keep beds full and census numbers up, much is compromised. Which in bad Nursing Homes such as this, residents were placed wherever there was an open bed. Regardless of compatibility.

Back to Doris, whenever you worked, you had to always watch out for her. Especially if she wasn't in her room. She was like a mischievous child, If she wasn't within your eyesight, she was probably somewhere doing something that she wasn't supposed to be doing.

One day I was sitting at the nurses' station doing some charting and talking to Nechelle, the other Nurse who was working that day, and there came Doris talking loudly to her self and walking back and forth.

"Doris, sit down somewhere and cut out all of that racket!" I yelled. I went back to my charting.

She kept rambling loud about something as usual. We tried to ignore her.

A resident was sitting near the nurses' station, Mrs. Franklin, quiet and really sweet. She never bothered anyone.

All of a sudden, I hear a loud screeching noise, its Doris pulling herself a chair from the dining room. She pulls her chair next to Mrs. Franklin.

"ok, if you're going to sit there, be nice," I say.

'ok, nursie" she says innocently.

The calm before the storm, and before anyone could stop her, she stood up, bent over, pulled the wheelchair of Mrs. Franklin away from the wall, bent down, lifted it from the front, and dumped Ms. Franklin out of the chair. Doris then ran down the hall to her room,......as she always did.

Nechelle and I ran to Mrs. Franklin to make sure she was okay. Two of us lifted the chair upright and checked Mrs. Franklin to make sure that she was okay, she was. I looked her skin over for any scratches, bruises, or redness. I checked her head for any lumps or bumps, she seemed to be okay. I think she was more startled and frightened than anything else, she cried like a baby. It took us a while to reassure her and to calm her down. Everyone was upset with Doris. She had probably propped a chair against her door. She always did this; the chair was easily pushed away from the door, and if that didn't work, we could enter the adjoining room to get in and talk to her. I went into her room, and she immediately started hitting and swearing at me.

I stared at her until she stopped.

"Are you calm now?"

"yes, honey," she said.

"now why did you do that to Mrs. Franklin? Dump her out of her chair. You could have really hurt her."

"I'm sorry I won't do it again." She says.

We left her alone in her room. She returned to the nurses' station a short time later, naked and dancing around, per the usual.

"that's a hoochie-coochie dancer," one of the male residents exclaimed with a big smile on his face.

One of the CNA'S grabbed a towel and started "shooing" her back to her room.

"put some clothes on, you loose woman, have some decency about yourself." Says the same cna.

The way that the CNAs handled her was a completely different matter from the way the Nurses dealt with her. They would usually do something to her. I just didn't know what it was. I'd just see her running down the hall away from one of them one minute. Then her chasing after one of them the next.

Of course, the cna's would deny that they were doing anything wrong to her.

It was tough getting past one thing that Doris did ! when she was always doing something new!

One Sunday morning, one of the CNAs, Monica, wasn't paying attention and was sitting half asleep. Doris quietly crept up next to her and slapped her silly! Doris then ran off.

(it was funny to me, but not to Monica)

I believe that this was not random, Doris had her moments. Who knows, Monica may have done something to her another day and Doris hadn't forgotten.

Anyway, after that slap Doris took off running, Monica quickly jumped up and was fast on Doris' heels. I jumped up just as quickly to intervene.

Monica is about to lose her job and her CNA license.

I caught Monica just in time, she was pissed!

I convinced her to let it go, this wasn't worth losing her lively hood over.

Besides, I didn't care too much for Monica, she was lazy, and you barely got any work out of her. It was hard for me to feel sorry for her.

I suspect that Monica will get Doris back the first chance she gets, when no one is around, of course.

Fast forward, it's Saturday morning, and I have 16 long hours to work today. I was working with Nechelle again.

It can be hard finding the right fit for two nurses to work together daily. I was the one newly hired, so I had to learn to be tolerable in making this work relationship work.

Overall, I didn't mind working with Nechelle. She was brash, loud, rude, unprofessional at times, always eating in the nurses' station, always burping, and could generally be quite annoying. However, she was one of the best nurses I knew, and underneath it all, she knew her shit. You just had to get to know her.

We were both working 16-hour shifts this particular Saturday. Doris was in one of her moods. When she was like this, we had to frequently check on her roommate. I had spoken to my supervisor at least twice regarding the idea that Doris have a private room or at least put her in a room with someone who was alert and could talk. I was told that Doris couldn't afford a private room and that there were no other female beds available. I contend that Doris should not be in a room with a person who cannot speak nor defend herself. All the nurses offered their opinion regarding possible room changing options.

Doris was just too unstable and aggressive, and everyone, including all of the managers, knew it.

Doris' roommate was Ms. Mamie, who didn't speak, was contracted, and had multiple medical problems.

If this were another place and time and Ms. Mamie could walk, and talk, I imagine she and Doris would have physically fought- constantly, as Ms.Mamie was actually pretty mean herself.

Ms. Mamie might not have been in her right mind and couldn't make her needs known, but she could fight like you wouldn't believe.

I often wondered if part of the reason she was so mean was because of the way she was treated by the nursing assistants. The care she was/was not receiving from our facility. After all, we did have the reputation of being the worst Nursing Home in the city.

None of the cna's liked caring for her because she fought so badly. When she had to be fed, she would hit you while you fed her. When she had to be bathed and changed; she usually hit you while you did this.

Anything you tried to do for her, she fought you; and when I say the care that she was/was not receiving I mean that because she was so mean the nursing assistants did the most minimal for her. When they did do anything, they tried to get it over with as quickly as possible. This offered her minimal contact with people and when she did have contact it was painful. This is the case with many nursing home residents like Ms. Mamie. It also didn't help that her contractures were really bad, and it hurt her to be moved unless the cna's were extra gentle with her, and none of them were.

Anyway, they wouldn't change the room assignments, she was Doriss' roommate, and that was that.

Nechelle and I are sitting in the nurses' station drinking coffee, gossiping, and doing paperwork; we were hoping for a quiet Saturday afternoon.

I sshhh Nechelle, "I thought I heard yelling."

We listen. Nothing. We start to talk again.

There it was again… I thought I heard yelling, I couldn't be sure.

"I'll be right back," I said.

I checked around for the sound.

I walked down the hall.

there it was again

It seemed to be coming from Doris' room.

"Oh shit!"

I rushed in, and there was Doris standing over Ms. Mamie, hitting her in the chest and yelling in her face.

Ms. Mamie was moaning and crying.

I immediately rushed towards the two of them. As I did so, Doris pushed past me and ran away.

I ran to Ms.Mamie and leaned over to comfort her, and to my surprise, she let me.

I just kept talking to her.

"You're ok, you're ok."

I glanced over her body and looked for signs of injury. I didn't see any. This wouldn't change the paperwork that I would have to do. I was so upset with Doris; I had had it with her. I went back to the nurses' station and I told Nechelle everything that had happened.

Where was Doris hiding? I found her in the TV room, sitting innocently as if she hadn't done anything. I had a CNA keep an eye on her while I made some phone calls and did paperwork because of this incident. As I sat making my calls and charting, I told Nechelle that come Monday management is going to have to do something about those two in a room together, or I'm calling "State!"

The State (as they call it) is who you call (anonymously if you like) when you have a complaint regarding a facility. An incident that you believe requires an outside investigation. They have the power to motion for the closing of a facility.

It's sad, but most owners of Nursing Homes don't have a clue as to what really happens behind their doors. They only know what is being told to them, and usually, that is not the truth. (We can talk more about that in another chapter.) Managements job is, in my opinion, to hide the truth. To dress everything up so that it "appears" to be a certain way. The last thing that they want to do is to lose money, and no facility is going to lose money because of our opinions of safety; even if it was the right thing to do.

Out of nowhere, an idea came to me from something I had recently seen on a science channel.

I told Nechelle about it. She laughed and thought that it could work. As soon as we finished our paperwork, we jumped into action.

I got some hot water from the faucet, and I mixed salt into it. I then took a large 60cc syringe with a large 18g needle. Nechelle concocted the same preparation. Hot salt water!

I went back to the TV room where she was sitting. She wasn't there. The cna was still sitting there watching TV, she said that she hadn't realized that Doris was gone.

Nechelle and I searched for Doris.

We found her in one of the other residents' rooms. We slowly approached her, she looked up and saw us coming, she took off running. She ran straight for her own room.

Perfect!

We followed her. I did all of the talking. I started telling Doris that she would have to be punished for what she had done to Ms. Mamie. She started cursing at us, yelling at us. She jumped up to charge at us. We pulled our arms from behind our backs and revealed the syringes. She stopped. I don't think she knew what to think. I think it then came to her.

"I don't want a shot, don't you give me a shot!" she yelled.

We told her that she wouldn't be getting a shot but that she was getting something much worse than a shot. We told her that our syringes contained acid and that we were going to use it to burn her skin off. She listened as we both said to her that she should apologize to Ms. Mamie for hitting her. She started to cry, *it was fake, she always cried when she got into trouble.*

We followed her, syringes out as she walked to Ms. Mamie's bedside, and apologized.

"I'm sorry, ma'am I won't hit you again, accept my apology please!"she said.

We were actually surprised that she did this. She had never apologized for anything before.

It didn't matter; we were determined to scare her for what she had done to Ms. Mamie.

We yelled at her, "Prepare to be punished!"

Nechelle and I started to shoot her with our hot salt-water concoction. She screamed and cried, "It burns, it burns, my skin is falling off."

Nechelle and I kept shooting her with the water until our syringes were empty.

We then ran out of the room and to the nurses' station. We laughed until we were crying. We couldn't stop laughing. We could hardly sit still.

It didn't take Doris long to get over this.

A short time later, Doris came running out of the room yelling and looking for "those bitches!"

She was showing anyone and everyone who would look at her, her skin, and how it was burned and falling off because of the acid.

All the nursing assistants looked confused because they didn't know what she was talking about. One of them looked at her arms and legs and told her that she didn't see anything wrong with her skin.

"Go and have one of the nurses to look at you." She told her.

As she walked away, I heard one of the nursing assistants say to her "well it would serve you right for always being mean!"

As she walked toward the Nurses station, she spotted us and started yelling. She ran at us. Nechelle and I started laughing again until she ran INTO the nurses' station trying to get to us.

"you bitches, whores…." She yelled. She had caught us off guard by actually coming into the nurses' station. We almost fell out of our chairs running from her. We ran out of the nurses' station laughing. We all ran around and around, a circle in and out of the nurses station. All of the CNAs were laughing. They didn't know what to make of things. She finally stopped inside the Nurses station and started throwing all of our charts and papers all over the place. The CNA's finally grabbed her and sat her down. She rambled on about acid on her skin. The cna's kept asking us what we had done. Nechelle and I never admitted to anything. We laughed every time we thought about it. Doris might have been confused but she tried all day to get a hold of Nechelle and me. She finally seemed to give up. Much later that evening, she came to the nurses' station and asked us ever so sweetly why we had burned her with acid.

" Because you hit someone, and that wasn't nice," we told her.

She simply stated "oh" and walked away. It was a good trick to keep her in line. Especially on the weekends when there was no management around. We couldn't dare do something like that during the week. Either way, this worked for a long time. We would just flash a syringe at

Doris, and as my daddy would say, she'd "straighten up and fly right," and off she would go running promising not to do something again.

We were able to control Doris for quite some time with this little act.......... quite some time.

Sins of Nurses

"Death is not the greatest loss in life. The greatest loss is what dies inside us while we live."

-Norman Cousins

Chapter 12

I ALMOST KILLED HIM

I was working at this particular nursing home for the first time through an agency. This meant that I didn't know any of the residents and that I didn't know any of the nurses.

UUUgghh!

Where is the MAR?

Where is the cardex?

I found them and looked at them. The cardex was outdated and of no use to me. The MAR showed me that I would be passing lots of medications at 9am and 1pm, and there was a shit load of diabetics to check around 11am right before lunch. There were also many treatments to do. As usual, I would do the best that I could and get through this day with my sanity and license intact; and hopefully, without any falls happening. I would have to rely on the nursing assistants to get the medications to the right residents; in theory, they should be able to help me identify who was who; especially since none of the residents wore name bands in this facility. There were two nurses on this floor, myself and another nurse.

It turns out that she hadn't been to this facility before, either.

This was going to be a long day.

I had hoped that I would be able to rely on whomever the other nurse was to help me through my day. That wasn't going to happen.

As our day started, we were both barely able to get our medications passed to the residents. We both seemed to have lots of problems. Half of the medicine that I was to give went right into the trash still crushed in applesauce.

"ugggh!" this sucks.

One after the other, I tried to coax and beg the residents to take their medications, no luck. They don't know me.

"ugggh!" this really sucks.

I tried to enlist the help of the nursing assistants whenever I could. This med pass was overwhelming. No one can understand the pressure of it all, except another nurse. There are all of these critical medications that have to be given for hypertension, seizures, heart problems, diabetes!!! Most of the residents will not take them. There are many reasons why a resident won't take their medication. It might be that they don't like the taste, others don't want it because they just don't want it, others are simply confused and have some form of dementia.

The reality is that no one really cares about how residents feel. Doctors just prescribe and want the resident to have the medication.

What should a nurse do?

Families know that they need the medication and want them to have it, usually by any means necessary and will say things like

"Oh, just squeeze her cheeks, and she'll take it."

"We hold her nose at home."

"I don't care how she gets it; you know she could die without it!" Residents just know that they don't want any part of taking medicine.

All of these thoughts are going through my head as I am trying to give this medicine.

Mid-thought, Nancy (the other nurse that I am working with) comes into the room. She closes the door and starts going on and on.... It's not fair, it's overwhelming. I'm half-listening to her. I just agree with whatever she is saying.

"Oh my god, oh my god." I hear her say.

I keep trying to get my patient to take his medication.

I'm deep in thought.

She keeps rambling.

As she is talking, I notice that her voice is trembling. I look up and see that she has tears in her eyes.

"Are You ok? "

She shakes her head, "No."

"What's going on?" I ask her

She looked me in the eyes, trying to decide if she wanted to trust me. She doesn't know me, and I don't know her.

She then swears me to secrecy and makes me promise that I won't repeat what she is about to tell me.

"Ok, what's up?

I'm wondering what has happened.

She goes on to tell me that she has only been a nurse for 2 years and that she has just made her first nursing error.

I had heard other nurses talk about making huge mistakes. I had been a nurse for over 10 years and had never made any major mistakes. I'm lucky.

Ultimately, I guess we all think that it can never happen to us. I'm just listening to her.

She began to blurt it out.

"I've just made a med error. I gave the wrong medication to a resident."

Okay, there, she said it, no turning back.

"Are you sure?" I ask.

"Yes," she says.

"Why don't you just go and talk to one of the managers?" I ask her.

"I don't want to do that just yet," she says.

"Well what is it that you want me to help you with," I ask

"Just do me a favor and help me look at this MAR."

"Ok, give me a second, " I tell her.

I get to her cart and she starts to explain how the error happened.

I glance over at the clock.

She explains that she went into a room to give medicine and that there were two Hispanic male residents there.

She says she introduced herself.

Neither said anything.

She says they both were alert and staring at her but didn't seem to be verbal.

She says she asked the bed A resident, "Good morning sir, are you, Mr. Rivera?" He nodded, yes.

She gave him his medication, no problems there.

She then went to bed B resident to give him medication.

"Good morning Mr. Gonzalez, I have your medicine."

She started to give him his medicine. At that moment, the nursing assistant walked into the room and quietly asked, "Did you say, Mr. Gonzalez?"

"Yes"

"That's not Mr. Gonzalez, that's Mr. Rivera."

She says she looked at her with a confused face and stated that she had just asked Mr. Gonzalez his name, and he said that he was Mr. Rivera.

She says the CNA then asked her, "He actually said that he was Mr. Rivera? "

"Well, no, but he acknowledged that he was when I asked him. "

"I know what you are saying, but if you ask him if his name is Mr. Cat, he will say yes to you." The CNA said.

To prove her point, she did just that

"Hello, Sir, how are you today?" Said the Bed A resident.

"Fine," he replied.

"Is your name Mr. Cat?"

"Yes." He replied.

"That was a close call, huh, nurse." the CNA says.

"Ok, thanks; let me look at my MAR again." She says she told the CNA.

She says she immediately turned around and went to her cart to get the correct medicine for Mr. Rivera, which she then gave to him. It was then that she looked at the correct medication for Mr. Gonzalez. It was nothing close to the medication that she had just given him.

"Let's look," I tell her.

We look at the MAR to see the correct medications that should have been given to Mr. Gonzalez.

Maybe it will be that she gave him nothing too serious. At least I was hoping, for her *sake, maybe most of the medicines that she had given him were vitamins and iron or something.*

But no, they weren't. They were mostly blood pressure and heart related.

"Well, you gotta talk to one of the nursing managers here." I tell her.

But first, let's at least get some vitals, and then we'll call the doctor and speak to a manager."

"There is a house supervisor here, let me find a number for you."

"Nooooooo, I can't do that!" she exclaimed.

"Do what?" I asked.

"Any of it, I can't, I can't chance my license for this."

"It's just a med error; you won't lose your license for a mistake," I tell her.

She goes into the room and checks his vital signs. She says their normal.

I ask her again, "would you like me to call for you?"

"No, I don't want to call anyone just yet." She says.

"Well, what then do you want to do? "

"I want to just watch him and see what happens."

"Then why did you tell me if you were just going to watch him?"

"Because I had to tell someone, and I think I can trust you."

I shake my head.

I don't know, maybe he'll be fine, I think to myself.

Then I ask her, "Does Mr. Gonzalez have any heart or blood pressure problems?"

"I'm not sure," she replied.

"You need to look up his medical history and watch him closely. I really hate that you told me this!"

She apologizes. "I'm sorry, but I just can't report this."

I head down the hall to finish giving medicine to my patients. When I'm done, I meet her back at the nurses' station. We go back to the patient's room to assess him. He seems to be ok. His vital signs are still normal.

The CNA comes into the room and says that she is going to get both Mr. Rivera and Mr. Gonzalez up and out of bed in a few minutes.

We talk some more then head to the nurses' station.

She decides that she will call the supervisor regarding the medication error.

The nursing supervisor calls to our unit to check on us, since we were both agency. I listen as she starts to tell her that she gave the wrong medication but just at that moment, we hear through the facilities paging system that there is a medical emergency on one of the other floors. The nursing supervisor leaves and tells the nurse to fill out an incident report and that she will return in a few.

"Make sure you monitor the resident and don't forget to call the doctor."

I saw the supervisor run down the hall to the medical emergency. I went back down the hall to do some of my work that was piling up. I saw her about an hour later and asked her how things were going. She said that the resident's vital signs were still good and that he was sitting in the day room watching television. I asked her what the doctor said. She confided in me that she hadn't called and that her intent was to watch him closely since he seemed to be okay.

We had about 2 hours before our shift was to end, and she thinks that he will be okay.

"What are you going to tell the supervisor if she asks you about the incident report and the call to the doctor ?"

She said that she hadn't figured that part out yet. I didn't say anything.

Just then, one of the nursing assistants comes to the nurses' station and says that Mr. Gonzalez is behaving strangely. We both jump up. When we arrive to the TV room, he is slightly slumped and appears to be a bit lethargic. We call his name and check his vital signs again, they seem stable enough. Admittedly, he does appear to be lethargic. I think she (we) are taking a big chance with him. I then tell her that she needs to not take any more chances and to send him to the emergency room. She reluctantly agrees that she will send him to the emergency room. I help her start the paperwork to transfer him to the emergency room.

Nancy calls the House supervisor and lets her know that she is sending a resident to the hospital for altered mental status and lethargy.

The supervisor gives an ok for this.

EMS arrives a short time later and Nancy tells them that she isn't sure what is wrong with him. That there appears to be an altered mental status and lethargy. They check his vital signs and find that he seems to be stable. They take him to the local hospital. Our shift is to end in a few minutes. We don't discuss what has happened. The nurses' station phone rings and it is the supervisor calling to check on the patient that she gave the wrong medication to. I listened as Nancy told her that she hadn't made a mistake after all, she only thought that she had. She ended her phone call with the supervisor. I don't think the supervisor gave it another thought. I don't think that she initially knew that Mr. Gonzalez was the resident who had gone to the hospital.

I had mixed feelings the duration of my shift. I was glad that Mr. Gonzalez was safely sent to the hospital for observation. Our relief nurses came and we gave report. I know that she never told anyone other than me what had happened. As our shift ended, I hurried out of the building. I was standing at my car when Nancy caught up with me.

"Hey, are you working here tomorrow?" She asked me.

"Yes, I am, are you?"

"No," she replied. She lingered for a minute as if she wanted to say something more. I continued to put my things in the trunk of my car. I didn't say anything. She finally blurted out

"I can't afford to lose my license, please don't say anything!"

I didn't look up at her, and neither did I say anything.

She stood silently for a while and then she walked away. I got into my car and I drove away. I couldn't sleep that night; I hoped that Mr. Gonzalez would be okay, and if by chance, he was not, what should be my next move.

I came in the next morning. The staffing person had placed me on the same unit that I had worked the day before. I walked down the hall to Mr. Gonzalez's room. He wasn't back. I asked about him, but no one seemed to know anything. Maybe he was fine. The other nurse that I was working with stated that she had called the hospital for an update, and the hospital stated that he would probably be released sometime in the next 24 hrs.

I hoped so. My day went by uneventfully. The supervisor approached me at one point and asked me if I knew anything about Nancy, giving the wrong medications to Mr. Gonzalez.

I drew a blank.

She went on to say that, the nurse that I had worked with on yesterday mentioned a medication error and was to fill out an incident report. That the resident had indeed gone out to the hospital but that there was no incident report or note regarding her medication error.

I tried not to look guilty.

"No, I don't know anything about anything like that."

She stared at me, really stared. She then said to me,

"You weren't sitting with her when she called me?"

"I thought I heard your voice in the background saying something to her."

I said that I vaguely recalled her calling but that I didn't recall the conversation.

"You don't recall her stating that she gave the wrong medication to a resident?" She continued to stare at me.

"No, I was really busy at that time. I really don't remember her conversation with you."

She then asked, "Did she say anything to you about the resident she sent to the hospital?"

I lied and stated that she had only said that he was lethargic and behaving strangely. She stared at me.

"Okay, "she said.

She knew that I knew more. Nurses for all of their backbiting behaviors still have a loyalty to one another with some things.

I wasn't going to say anything, and I don't want to think about the choice that I would have had to make had Mr. Gonzalez died. I went back to doing my work.

I kept working and counting down the time until my shift ended. The end of my shift couldn't get here soon enough. I couldn't wait to get out of that building. Just as I was leaving at around 4pm, an ambulance was arriving. I stood for a second and watched as the doors of the ambulance opened, I looked inside. It was Mr. Gonzalez.

I sighed with relief. I never saw Nancy again.

Sins of Nurses

"Every man has his secret sorrows the world knows not and often times we call him cold when he is only sad."

-Henry Wadsworth Longfellow

Chapter 13

DEFEATED

He was sitting in a wheelchair when his two daughters brought him in. One of the daughters simply walked to the nurses' station with some paperwork and handed everything to me. I glanced over them. I had already gotten his chart and admission paperwork from Joan in admissions. I took the papers anyway and put everything into his chart. I then directed the woman to the business office. She stated that her sister was already in the business office but that she would head there just in case they needed something from her. Just before she turned to head to the business office, she looked at me in a matter-of-factly kind of way and said,

"Please call us only if he dies."

I look into her eyes. She doesn't blink.

The daughter went on to say that, they did not want to receive calls for anything otherwise.

I can't say that I was too taken aback by this statement. Families dump so-called "loved ones" into Nursing homes every day. They pretend that they will be back very soon. They rarely return. Once every few months, if that.

At least, she was honest. Most families think it and don't say it.

She continued to talk. Her tone became somewhat angry. Her voice trembled a bit, "He is a pedophile, he molested my sister and me as children, and we are only doing what we have to do in the eyes of God."

I couldn't believe that the daughter was saying this in front of everyone. It was as if she wanted everyone to know and to hate him as much as she apparently did.

"We have forgiven him, but we have not forgotten." She said as she walked away with her chin up and back straight. "Please make sure you stop by admissions before you leave so that they may make a note of this," I whisper to her.

I felt as if I should say something more, but nothing came to mind. I guess there isn't much to say when you are caught off guard with something like this. I didn't want to insult her with something corny like, " I'll be praying for you and your family." Or "God heals all things." It felt too personal a thing to make any further mention.

I let her walk away.

Moving forward, this then set the tone as to the way almost everyone would treat Bill, the nursing assistants, to be more specific.

Bill's most major medical diagnosis was that he had cancer, metastatic cancer, he also had a huge bedsore covering most of his butt. Bill was a large man, considered morbidly obese. He couldn't walk, nor could he support his body weight. The doctors had given him a poor prognosis.

To make matters, worst Bill was mean and rude as hell most of the time. His behavior was a problem. We, the nurses, had several conversations on how we could counter this situation. He seemed to be disrespected by most of the nursing assistants. We needed the support of management to support us if we found that a CNA was disrespectful or unprofessional toward Bill.

If the managers didn't have our backs, then it would be useless for any Nurse to say anything to any CNA.

We started with the things that were out of control. The name-calling by certain CNAs. It was a vicious circle of events. Either he would say something to them and set things off, or they would say something to him, and it would set him off.

"You cocksucker, get out of my room." Says Bill

"Shut up, you piece of shit," yells the CNA.

Carmen, Carmen! You can't do that! I pull her to the side.

"You nigger bitch!" he yells

"White trash," she yells back.

"Carmen, I really don't want to write you up, but this name-calling has to stop, you know that," I tell her

"Ok, Nurse, but did you hear what he called me?" I did, and I'm going to speak to him.

I go into Bill's room. "Good morning Bill."

"I hate that bitch," he says.

"I know, but we gotta stop the name-calling, and that has to go both ways. Them with you, You with them." I tell him.

"Close the door on your way out." He says.

I shake my head, leave the room, closing the door behind me.

We just couldn't seem to come up with a resolution to this situation yet.

He seemed to hate all of the CNAs, and they hated him right back. The nursing assistants were to take care of him in pairs. For two reasons, one was because of his and their accusations to one another and two for back safety reasons. He was so large that it usually took two people to turn and hold him so that the nurse could change the dressing to the wound on his butt. It was a daily fight amongst the cna's as to whose rotation that it was to care for him. It was difficult for everyone involved. Each day it became more and more evident that this was a toxic environment.

The psychiatrist had diagnosed Bill as being schizophrenic and bipolar. His mental illnesses contributed, in part, to the reason that he was placed into our facility. Bill had been living alone and just wasn't able to adequately care for himself anymore. He was aware that he had Cancer and chose to forego any treatments. At home, he stated that he had had trouble walking, so he used a wheelchair or stayed in bed. I believe that he stayed in bed more than he was out of bed. He said that he had friends who went to the store for him and that he had a caregiver for 6 hours of the day who cooked and prepped meals for him. Since his arrival at our facility, Bill stayed in bed 100% of the time. He refused to get out of it. It was this lying in bed and lack of movement, not to mention no bathing that had caused Bill to develop a horrible decubitus (or bedsore) to his butt. This was not something that could be easily fixed; he required IV antibiotics, daily nursing care, and TIME. He needed nurses and CNAs to assist him daily. He required assistance to get into his chair, to turn, to hower…anything! Whatever the task, it would require 2-3 people to accomplish it. This was difficult, especially since no one liked him. At times he would hit and punch to keep anyone from touching him. This was unlike most of the other residents who wanted our help.

Maybe the real reason for his anger was in the accusations made by his daughter, I don't know.

In taking care of Bill, the only advantage that we had over him was that he liked to eat. He had a trust fund account in which he received deposits regularly. With his money, he would order fast food from any local spot, which would deliver. Bill loved his food, he loved to eat, and it showed.

As I said, he was a big man; he was well over 6′2, and he probably weighed almost 400lbs. Keeping his weight under control was hard, especially since he didn't see it as a problem. With him being so big, it required two CNAs to take care of him. There was only one nursing assistant who could take care of him alone and quickly. It was from Carl. We were very short-staffed today, so I was going to have to depend on Carl.

The problem was that Bill hated Carl and that feeling was mutual. Whenever you went into the room to do anything for him and Carl was with you, it became a war. The name-calling was terrible. He would call Carl "nigger," "ape" and any demeaning names he could think of. Carl would then call Bill "pedophile" "child molester" "fat asshole" and anything derogatory he could think of, in return. I came in one day in the middle of one of these wars. I had to ask Carl to step out of the room. He didn't want to but he did.

"And stay out!" Bill yelled to Carl who simply gave him the middle finger.

Bill looked at me and began yelling and hurling insults.

"You cow!"

"You're fucking ugly! "

"You whore!" He went on and on.

I sat down in the chair near his bedside until he tired of calling me names and stopped.

I then mustered all of the compassion I could gather.

"Are you done?" I ask.

"Have I ever done anything to you, ever called you out of your name?" I ask.

He thought about it and finally replied.

"No"

I then asked him if he would like a cup of coffee. We all knew that he loved coffee. Luckily, for me, it was a Saturday morning, and I had some time to make a fresh pot.

Even if I hadn't had any time, I would have made time this particular morning. I had to do a 16-hour shift and I wasn't up for all of the fighting between Bill and the CNAs. Once calm, Bill seemed to open up to reasonable conversation with me.

"Would you like me to order you something from one of your take out menus?" I ask.

"No harm in that," he says.

I tell him that I will do this after I've changed his dressing. He agrees, and then to my surprise, he started talking to me. He began to tell me that he knew that everyone on the floor hated him. I hated to admit it, but there was some truth to his thoughts.

I assured him that that was not true.

He didn't seem to believe me.

He stated that he couldn't change the things that he had done or what he was. He couldn't change anything about his life. He seemed very remorseful.

I just listened to him.

I had made him a cup of coffee and had given it to him.

I listened for as long as I could.

I hated to stop him, but I really couldn't stay any longer. I then reminded him that I needed to change the dressings on his butt and that if he let me change them, I would try not to bother him too much today and that I would keep everyone else from bothering him as much as I could.

"and I'll order your food!" I tell him.

He agreed.

I felt that I had made a small connection with him.

I then had to tell him that we were short-staffed today and that I would have to have Carl to help me, but that I would make sure that Carl didn't insult him or call him any names. He reluctantly agreed. I left out of his room and asked Carl if I could talk to him. I explained that although Bill's family had said those things about him, he was going to have to stop the insults and unprofessional behavior while caring for Bill. I told him that after it was all said and done, Bill was still a patient and a resident in our facility. It was his home and not ours and that if he wanted to keep his job it was going to have to stop today. I tried to say it in such a way that I wasn't implying that I would get him fired but that the wrong person might overhear him, and then he could possibly lose his job.

You have to tread very lightly when you are speaking and performing teachable moments with CNA's.

Carl made it very clear that he didn't think that the facility would ever fire him ! under any circumstance.!

He was very arrogant, yet he was probably right. Everyone loved him. The facility needed him, and they thought he could do no wrong. This mentality in most facilities fuels abuse because when cna's are well-liked and trusted, it is tough for a Nurse to prove that they have done anything wrong. They simply don't believe you. They don't want to believe you.

"Who Carl, you're mistaken!"

"I've never known Carl to behave in such a way."

The girl in the staffing office knew that she could depend on Carl. Especially when she was in a bind and needed someone at the last minute. Carl was it. He was invaluable, and he rarely let the facility down, he would work double shifts when and if they asked him to. He would also stay over to help if they needed him to. Facilities love nursing assistants like this, especially male nursing assistants.

Either way, Bill, Carl, and I had to get through this process of performing his dressing change. Well, It helped that Carl and now Bill had a decent relationship with me.

Carl agreed that he would simply assist me and not call names or disrespect Bill while he was in the room helping. We went into Bill's room, and soon as their eyes locked and Carl's mouth showed a smirk, it sent Bill into attack mode. The name-calling, insults, and fighting began. Before I could diffuse things, Carl quickly grabbed Bill's arms and snatched him onto his side. "Come on Nurse, change the dressing, I don't have all day to be in here fighting with him!" Bill knew that he was no match against Carl's strength. Carl held him forcibly; I had to admit that he was using unnecessary roughness to hold Bill over.

I hurried and haphazardly got the dressing change done as fast as I could, which wasn't fast enough for any of us.

"I'm done." I finally say.

I tell Carl to ease up and to relax his hold.

Carl looked at me with irritation and did just that!

He simply let go of him. Bill flopped onto his back.

"You asshole!"

"You prick!"

Carl turned and walked out of the room, sweating, and still cursing *about not helping me later.*

I was hot, tired, and sweating.

I turned my attention to Bill; his pale skin had turned fire red, and he was sweating from the stress of all of this; I thought that I saw frustration, anger, and even helplessness. I looked into his eyes, and a few tears rolled down his face. He yelled, "Get out!"

My eyes locked onto his.

He simply looked defeated. There was a war inside of him, in his body, and his mind....his life. And there was the war we inflicted upon him. I looked away. I walked out of the room. I didn't report Carl

"If he has a bedsore, it's generally not the fault of the disease, but of the nursing."

-Florence Nightingale 1859

Chapter 14

A BED SORE

Residents in a Medicaid or Medicare certified Nursing home have certain rights and protections per state and federal law. One of these protections is that a resident who cannot turn or move him or herself should be turned every two hours. This turning is what will keep blood flowing and circulating to skin areas and prevents skin breakdown and resulting bedsores (or pressure ulcers).

That is if these things are done and done correctly.

A bed sore or pressure ulcer is definitely a reflection of the level of care given or not given to a patient; it is a reflection of everyone involved....from the CNA, to the Nurse, the managers, and even the Physician. The prevention of bedsores should be a goal of everyone involved; and it typically is. Many policies and manuals in a nursing home reflect the need to prevent bedsores. But that's all they are, pieces of paper. The real prevention is in the Nurses' and CNA's ' ability to work together. A good working relationship is critical in being able to accomplish and prevent a Bedsore. Especially if a resident has been identified as being at risk for skin break down.

Since the nursing assistant will usually see reddened skin or a bed sore first, it is their job to relay this information to the nurse in a timely manner.

In most facilities, there are policies that require nurses to look at the body of all the residents that they are responsible for on their shower day. This is the most natural time to look them over from head to toe. It's usually easier said than done. The Nurse is going about her day and will have to stop and run to the shower to perform this head to toe assessment to assure that the resident has no reddened or broken skin.

In a better facility, the nurses are running to the shower rooms looking at skin between all of the things that they already do.

In many facilities, the nurses simply take the word of the CNA that the skin looks good. They then sign off that this skin check has been done.

Bedbound residents are the most vulnerable and susceptible to bedsores. Usually, the nursing assistants who are the laziest try to make sure these types of patients are on their assignment.

Because they won't bother them or call for assistance.

Ms. Gantt had been in our facility for about 6 weeks. She was a quiet woman who did not speak. Everything was done for her….. feeding, clothing, turning, toileting everything!

She had no family to speak of; I think there might have been a daughter who would come to the facility around Christmas time to visit her. One day there was a change in the assignments and Tameka one of the better nursing assistants came to me and said that she thought that I should look at Ms. Gantt's bottom. She went on to tell me that she had noticed a small hole on the butt of Ms. Gantt.

"You mean a red spot?" I asked her.

She replied, "No, it's an actual hole."

I found this hard to believe. These things always start with a reddened area. If it were a hole already, that would mean that a few people dropped the ball in her care. I went into the room with Tameka to look at her butt. Tameka turned her on her side while I looked. There it was, a hole; I measured it to be 1"x1" and about ½" in depth. It had a foul odor and was draining. I immediately called the doctor for orders. Her regular nurse was Rayma, who I was filling in for. There were orders to change her dressing every day and to turn her every 2 hours. I wondered how this was going to go. She had a nursing assistant who sucked, and although Rayma was very nice, she sucked as a nurse. Rayna had no backbone and behaved as if she were terrified of Madison, the regular CNA on her hall assignment. Some Nurses are like this. They are truly afraid of the CNA's. As well, they should be.

It's easier to laugh, joke, convince, plead and befriend them into doing their job rather than having a simple expectation that they would come to work, punch the clock, and then do the job that they are paid to do.

It must have been about a month later before I worked Rayna's assignment again. I passed the scheduled medications. Then I went to start my treatments and dressing changes. I started with Ms. Gantt. I asked Tameka to help me by holding her on her side while I changed her dressing. We got her turned over, and soon as she was turned, I smelled an awful stench. I started removing the old dressings. What I found underneath was terrible. There was no way that her dressings had been changed daily. There was no way that she was turned every two hours. Her bed sore size had tripled in size and appeared to have tunneling. I couldn't believe it. The TAR was still reading as if she had a small wound that only required a wet to dry dressing once a day. I knew that there were two regular nurses who took care of her daily. On the day shift and the other on the evening shift. This facility didn't have a wound care Nurse. The Nurses were it. I called the doctor to get updated wound care orders. He gave strict orders to change her dressings twice daily. The products used to treat her bedsore were changed as well. Strict orders were implemented to keep the pressure off of her wound and to make sure that she was turned frequently.

A turning schedule was placed on the wall at the head of her bed. It's like a clock with no hands.

This would allow anyone to ascertain if she had been turned and if she had been turned, in which direction she should be facing.

For instance, you would know that at 3pm, she should be facing the window at 5pm she should be on her back, and then at 7pm, she should be facing the door. There's a turn that happens every 2 hours.

Most of the time when you went into the room she was not in sync with the turn schedule. If you then asked her nursing assistant, "is Ms. Gantt current with the turn schedule?" Usually there was some kind of story and the story didn't change much.

It was usually the same.

"I've been turning her every 2 hours we are just off schedule by a few minutes."

Of course, you couldn't prove that this wasn't true. But deep down, you knew it. The CNA's knew that you couldn't prove or disprove whether the turn schedule that they presented was accurate. What we did know was that by the next month, her bedsore was the size of a person's fist, and it continued to have a foul odor.

Ms. Gantt eventually developed a septic infection. She was placed on IV antibiotics. She never complained of pain, she never said a word. No family ever came. They even ordered a special mattress. Another month went by….her wound continued to grow in size. The CNAs continued to insist that they were turning her as ordered. The Nurses insisted that the dressing changes were being done twice daily.

I don't think that the nurses were changing her dressings as they were ordered. When you are really busy and have much going on, doing your treatments fall to the bottom of your priority list. The next time I saw Ms. Gantt she was lifeless and pale, not resembling what she had been a few months prior. She remained on IV Antibiotics. The CNA's were reporting that her appetite was poor and that she was barely eating. Her wound continued to grow larger. She was eventually placed on hospice.

She died a short time later. They assume natural causes to be the reason.

Sins of Nurses

"An eye for an eye only ends up making the whole world blind."

-Gandhi

CHAPTER 15

FAMOUS LAST WORDS OF A CNA IN A BAD NURSING HOME

1. The nurse needs to learn some respect.

2. The nurse needs to learn how to talk to people.

3. You're lucky I even came to work.

4. I'm not working if she's working, I'm going home.

5. I'm doing this facility a favor.

6. I can just go home.

7. This is the reason I don't work day shift

8. I'm not about to keep answering his/her call light, I just left out of that room.

9. I'm not feeding him/her.

10. I know I wasn't supposed to be in that patient's room on my cell phone, but that was an important call.

11. I'm not cleaning him/her up again.

12. I wasn't sleeping.

13. If I were a nurse…

14. If we all say that we saw her do it…

15. Anybody could do what a nurse does.

16. The nurse needs to get laid.

17. Six more hours until I clock out.

18. The nurse needs a life!

19. The nurse needs a drink.

20. That's not my patient

21. That's not my hall.

22. I just gave him a bed bath instead.

23. I'm on my break.

24. I just got here.

25. I'm off the clock

26. I'm going to start working the night shift

27. I could be at my other job

28. I'm going to the Administrator about this assignment

29. I'm calling off tomorrow

30. If I didn't need this job!!

"It's a good thing people can't read my mind."

-R.L Green

Chapter 16

THOUGHTS OF A NURSE

1. These cnas' need to learn the meaning of respect.

2. The cnas' need to learn how to talk period.

3. You're lucky I came to work, as well.

4. I wish I could go home, also.

5. I'm doing this facility a favor, also!!

6. I wish I could just go home, also.

7. That is the reason I wish YOU didn't work day shift

8. I'm not about to keep answering his/her call light, I just left out that room and I'm not a cna

9. I'm not feeding him/her, I'm not a cna

10. How can a cna sit at the Nurses desk more than a nurse

11. I'm not cleaning him/her up again, it's your job

12. I never get enough sleep.

13. If I were a doctor!...

14. We all "really" saw her do it, and nothing happened.

15. Anybody could do what a nurse does except a cna.

16. I probably "do" need to get laid.

17. Thirteen more hours until I clock out.

18. I need a life.

19. I need a drink NOW!

20. I "really" don't care if you take this medicine.

21. If you ring that call light one more time.

22. I just medicated him for pain.

23. I've been here for 6 hours and haven't had a break.

24. I just got here.

25. I'm off the clock.

26. I'm going to start working the night shift

27. I need another job.

28. Illiterate, unprofessional, ignorant assholes!

29. Not today, oh no, not today!

30. Did I say I need a drink?

31. Yes! The DON just said that

32. Yes! The housekeeper just did that

33. Yes! Your Mom said that

"Get your facts first, then you can distort them as you please."

-Mark Twain

Chapter 17

CERTIFIED NURSING ASSISTANTS

I can almost pinpoint when the change happened. It was under the presidential reign of then former President Bill Clinton. The year was 1996. Welfare Reform Act. PRWORA According to Bill Clinton, this was to end welfare as we had come to know it. In a nutshell, the Act was going to force individuals who did not work, had not worked, and whom (a questionable number) did not want to work; to get jobs. Can you guess which job was pushed to the top of the list? Pay above minimum wage, quick training, employment stability, and a huge shortage?

Just what was needed for this population and what the government wanted.

Certified Nursing Assistants, better known as CNAs. I became a Licensed Practical Nurse in 1991 and between

1991-2001. I loved Nursing. Everyone respected one another and worked hard. Everyone respected the profession and recognized one another as professionals in the care of taking care of those who couldn't take care of themselves. By 1998, there was an explosive number of CNAs from the welfare to work reform act. There were people of all nationalities, male and female. Reluctantly, unwillingly and with great hesitation, they came into the hospitals and nursing homes. Initially, we welcomed them. We tolerated some of the unprofessional, uneducated, lackadaisical, and sometimes ignorant behaviors.

We were happy to have the help. Slowly, but surely this group fast learned that they were much needed. They could work many hours, and they might as well because there was no going back to welfare. They flowed into the hospitals and nursing homes in high numbers. The hospitals could afford to be more selective in whom they hired, they had fat pockets, and they remain particular to this day. They were careful enough to hire the individuals within this group who wanted to work, positive attitudes, those who truly wanted off welfare, and wanted to learn a different way to live and provide for their families. Hospitals were and still are very practical in this regard. The Hospitals tried to maintain their high standards of doing business. They did a great job, and for the most part, they still do. As time went on, the nurses in the hospitals set a standard and made an effort to teach and guide. There was ongoing training that would discuss appropriate language in the workplace, dress codes, behaviors and etiquette in caring for patients and addressing their families. Anyone who did not conform, i.e. loud, brash, rude, and unprofessional, was terminated. If you didn't quickly exhibit a certain work ethic, you didn't stay in the hospital long. You went elsewhere to work. Nursing homes accepted any "body" that was warm. Everyone knew it. There was, seemingly, no standard there. I take that back, the standard was and is "if you are a warm body, you can work, bad attitude included free of charge."

They came to the Nursing home with no intent to change. The sentiment was that there was no need to change. Instead of the Nursing home, adapting the same standard as the hospital, they lowered it for the sake of numbers. The CNAs didn't see the elderly as our loved ones, those who were helpless and depended on us. They mostly and simply saw people who, most of the time, needed "shit" to be cleaned from them. Hence, their "shitty" attitudes, and when I say their attitudes were "shitty," I am being conservative. Their ethic was almost non-existent. We quickly lost control and never regained it. Not to this day and its 2020.

There are many reasons why it's remained this way! Some nurses are simply afraid of CNAs. Some are too busy to micromanage the care when stacks of charts and charting need to be done with endless meaningless paperwork put in place to cover the facilities' best interests.

Some simply look the other way. If it's out of sight, then it's out of mind. I've spoken to countless nurses over the last 25 years and have told many, very casually, that I was writing a book and wanted their honest opinions, observations, and their real stories. I assured them that I would not mention their names. Under a cloak of confidentiality, I've been told that there are numerous reasons as to why they have chosen to stand by quietly concerning nursing assistants and issues in Nursing.

It seems that a lack of support from management is at the top of the list.

Another is that nothing is going to be done or changed regardless of what we Nurses say or do.

Another common answer is job security.

Another is fear of retaliation, retaliation from CNA's, from coworkers, fear from unit managers, from ADON's, DON's and even Administrators.

But then this is only half the equation of why Nurses tolerate the things that we do. Why then do the Owners, Administrators, and parties in management look the other way when they know that the minimum is being done?

My opinion would be that it is based on money. Residents are charged daily for Nursing home care. Nursing Homes tend to structure their care delivery systems around the governmental Medicare payment system. In plain English, charges made to the patients are tailored to the maximum amounts that can be charged. Thus the creation of an atmosphere of fraud.

Back to Nursing Assistants.

CERTIFIED NURSING ASSISTANTS =USELESS, LAZY AND I'VE ONLY MET A HANDFUL THAT I HAVE LIKED!

In my over 25-years/career in nursing. I can almost count the number of CNAs that I have liked and thought were good enough to care for anyone that I knew and loved. This is my truth and my experience. Some of you Nurses, and family members may feel differently, and that will be your experience.

CNAs are generally mean, manipulative, lazy, and unhappy people. Many of the ones that I have met shouldn't have (and currently shouldn't be) working in Nursing homes...they should be in someone's jail somewhere. Over the years, I have reported, and reported, and reported the abuses and perpetuations of nursing assistants again. No one cares! Not the Unit managers, Nursing supervisors, Directors, or Administrators. It would be too costly to fire the inadequate ones. Quite frankly, as of this date, 9/5/2019, I think that most nursing homes, 95% of them, would have to close their doors if they had to terminate all of the bad nursing assistants and hire new and competent ones. If a facility had a staff of 75 CNAs and were told that there are 75 truly good and hardworking

CNAs waiting to replace the lazy ones, they would probably only keep 9 or 10 of the ones they currently have on staff. The rest would have to go. Many, many nurses would agree with me. I imagine that some would not.

I've talked to countless nurses and they usually say that the reason they accept this behavior from the CNAs is that:

it is easier to go along with the CNAs rather than try to get them to do the work that is expected of them.

We're just tired of complaining and getting no results. We realized a while ago that complaining wouldn't do any good.

Some nurses are afraid of the CNAs.

Many of us agree that nursing assistants are a foul bunch.

I'm sure to get some opposition from "some" nurses regarding this issue but far more praise from the majority of the nurses because I'm speaking the truth regarding nursing assistants in the Nursing Home.

I guess every nurse has a different story to tell. I can only focus on my own. If there is a nurse somewhere who has a different experience, good for you. I only ask that those Nurses who have those great stories to tell regarding their cna's, please remember that this is my experience, not yours. Please have 10+years before you comment on what is truth or not truth regarding my accounts of cna's.

Nurses with longevity know what I am talking about. When you find a good CNA, you are lucky if you can keep them for any length of time. Usually they are run off by the bad CNAs or the politics of working in a nursing home.

What are the politics? Ok, take, for instance, each nursing assistant is responsible for eight patients each. Each might have four total care patients, patients that require that you feed them, dress them, bathe them…and that CNA would also have four other patients who need minimal to medium care. But when politics are involved, meaning who kisses up to the nurse or supervisor the most, the good nursing assistant might get six residents who are difficult and require lots of care and only one or two who can do anything for themselves. And that CNA, who is a lazy, loudmouth, might get six to seven minimal patients and only one to two total care patients. The good CNAs usually won't complain too much, which keeps them with the assignment that sucks.

In addition, when it comes to being run off, the lousy nursing assistants usually make them miserable, and they leave, or they begin to conform to the wrong way of doing things. I mean, what can you do when you work with four other people who hide in resident rooms and sleep, watch TV, talk on the cell phones, and try their hardest to do the barest minimum. Then there is you sticking out like a sore thumb, and guess what? When you stick out like that, people tend to notice you. Then what? The things that people want to ignore can't be ignored! Therefore, someone has to change, and many do. But in which direction?

There are some that continue to march and play to their own drum, they try to give their best every time that they work. I've met a few awesome CNAs, and I wish that I could name them, but it would have involved tracking them down and obtaining their consent.

Most CNAs who remember me know that I understood their plight. They knew that I got it and understood what they were going through. I have had many conversations over the years with many CNAs who wished that they could do better, but they can't because of the politics of Nursing homes. They might be faced with four to five other CNAs against them complaining and lying as if they were the problem. I knew exactly how they felt.

You know what partially inspired me to write this book? Some years ago, I was watching one of the court TV shows, I don't recall which one. But the show went something like this (to the best of my recall) there was a nurse who brought a nursing assistant to court and was suing her. I believe she had lost her job and was claiming that this CNA had created a stressful work environment. She said some other things that she was charging her with as well.

Anyway, as the case was presented I was out of my seat in amazement….yelling at the TV.

I could soooo relate to everything that this nurse was saying. It actually brought tears to my eyes. I remember that as the nurse was narrating the actions of the nursing assistant, the judge was in absolute disbelief

My impression was that the judge couldn't comprehend that these things could have happened as the Nurse was explaining the events.

That nurse her case because the things that she described were so outlandish and unbelievable to everyone in the courtroom.

But with tears in my eyes, I knew that everything that she had said was true.

I knew, and I understood.

I couldn't explain it to anyone why that case made me so emotional....it's kind of like the stories in this book. No one will believe that these things can be real or those unit managers, supervisors, directors; administrators can know of these things and look the other way. I wish I could scream it! They don't care...they really don't care. How can nurses go to work every day in nursing homes and do what we do and look the other way? We have no choice. We must come into that nursing home and do the very best that we can do with what we have. I have had many closed-door conversations with nurses about the nursing assistants and their behavior. We all agree that we are powerless. I'm not saying that there isn't a Nursing home somewhere, which has a **whole** team of competent, caring, hardworking nursing assistants. I am saying that in over 25 years and eight states later, I NEVER KNEW OF ONE!

*** Sins of Nurses ***

"Be who you are and say what you feel because those who mind don't matter, and those who matter don't mind."

- Bernard M. Baruch

Chapter 18

INAPPROPRIATE

It was going to be a long evening and an even longer night. It was only 5pm, and I was getting an admission. And to make matters worse, I was to work a double shift. 16 long hours! On at 3pm off at 7:30am.

I had to hurry and pass meds so that I could prepare for my admission.

What I knew was that it would be a black male, 31 years old, who was recovering from a sickle cell crisis. He had been in the hospital for over a week. It appears that they had finally gotten his pain under control and gotten rid of the swelling in his hands and feet.

He arrived, untimely as admissions do.

He arrived via an ambulance. I directed them down the hall, on the right, room 171. I glanced up at him. I did a double-take.

Wow, he was handsome

I quickly gathered all of my paperwork and headed down the hall to his room. The EMS guy was saying something to me. I half-heard it, I was admiring my new patient.

He sat up and simply moved from the gurney and into the bed. Once there, he placed his hands behind his head and crossed his legs; he wanted a response. I didn't entertain him.

At least not out loud

I introduced myself and let him know that I would be his Nurse throughout the night and until 7:30 tomorrow morning.

My night had just got exciting

I started my admission questions. I had already glanced at the 3008(the form sent by the hospital that enables you to admit the patient into your facility) sent over from the hospital. It gave a brief history and insight as to what he would need from us. Let's see, 31 years old, 6'4", and 210 lbs Sickle Cell crisis. He probably wouldn't be with us more than a few days, not sure why they even sent him to us.

Some of the history notes imply that he appeared to have a manipulative personality; we'll see.

He asked what kind of medication he would be on for his pain. He stated that he would like to have Injectable morphine but that he would take a couple of Lortab(narcotic pain pills) to "hold him over."

He stared at me, flashing a gorgeous smile the whole time. I tried not to stare, but he was so damned sexy; he knew it.

"Mr. Jones I need to grab some forms for you to sign, I'll be right back," I said.

I stood and adjusted my uniform.

His eyes were looking me up and down.

He was checking me out!

"you make sure and hurry back," he winked his eye at me.

I blushed a little.

I grabbed the papers and decided to call the doctor while I was there. The doctor gave me orders for the medications that he would need, this included a pain medication. He wouldn't be getting the morphine injection that he wanted, but he could have two Lortab now (maybe me later), and He would be getting that every 6hrs until the doctor saw him on Monday.

I walked back to his room and told him what the doctor had said and what medications he would have.

He looked at me and said, "I guess you are going to have to sit on my face or do something extra to make me feel better since I won't be getting my morphine shots."

I smiled and pretended to ignore him. I continued with my line of medical questions. "Do you have any other medical problems that I need to be aware of?"

"Did they tell you that I have severe eczema?"

"No." I stated, "It's not mentioned here."

"Well, I need that cream, its' called Eucerin. Do you think you have it here?" he asks.

"We'll come back to that."

"Could you stand up for me and take your clothes off, Mr. Jones? I just need to look at your skin as part of my admission assessment."

"Call me, Ken," He says.

"Do you have any surgical scars or skin issues other than eczema? KEN"

"You tell me." As he is taking off his clothing down to his underwear. He then stands up directly in front of me.

Lord, have mercy!! He was HOT

He had the lean, solid body of a swimmer or runner with a golden brown skin tone.

I could see signs of eczema to his upper body, back, and front. I made a notation of this.

He asks about the Eucerin cream again.

"We have it here, but you know that I have to get an order from the doctor to let you have it."

"Well, chop chop," He smiled and winked his eye.

I walked away, "asshole!"

"Glad to be one," he yells behind me.

I look back at him and smile, he licks his lips.

My shift seemed to be going smoothly despite dealing with this admission. It was now after 12 am, officially the night shift. There was only one nurse now and two CNAs for 40 residents.

The CNAs did what they usually do. Undressed all of the residents and put them to bed.

They then got pillows and blankets, went into the dayroom, and got comfortable for the night. I sat alone at the nurses' station. Charting. It was now 2am, and a call light rang.

"Could one of you ladies grab that light?' no response.

The CNAs continued to sleep. I look over at the call light and its room 171.

I jumped up, adjusted my uniform, threw on a little more lip gloss, and went down the hall to his room......... eagerly.

I hadn't stopped thinking about him since he stood in front of me, almost naked.

I get to his room, knocked and then, and entered.

"I'm glad you are still here," he says.

"I told you I would be here all night."

"How can I help you, Mr. Jones?" I say in my sweetest voice.

"My back is itching terribly. I can't stand it, and I need a pain pill."

"Let me go and get the pain medication, I'll be right back."

I return a short time later with his two Lortab. I told him that the doctor had approved the Eucerin cream but that it wouldn't be available for a few days. He said that he had a container in his bag. He pointed at the bag sitting in the corner.

I glanced into it, and there it was a full container.

"Ok, take your gown off, and I'll have the CNA to come in and put some on you."

"A CNA? Why not you!"

"Not my job, Mr.Jones."

"What sense does that make? YOU are in here right now, and I happen to know that you can't tell me that it's not your job! PATIENT CARE IS EVERYONES JOB.," he laughs.

I turned and grabbed a pair of gloves. I turned to approach him, and there he lay naked, uncovered, and with an erection. I was surprised, and yet I couldn't take my eyes off him.

"Mr. Jones!!!" I said.

He immediately started to apologize, "I'm sorry about this nurse." He covered himself.

"If you want me to put this cream on your back, don't try that again."

He apologized again and turned his back to me.

I began to apply the cream to his back. I kept seeing the image of his erection. I had started to rub firmly yet softly when he let out a moan. I continued to apply the cream to his back. He then turned from his back to his abdomen. He lay back, and without saying a word, he looked me in my eyes and grabbed my hand and placed it on his erection.

Beautiful

I moved my hand but continued to apply the cream to his body.

Slowly around his nipples, down the middle of his chest

I continue to apply the cream to his chest and abdomen. His erection returned. I didn't stop. I couldn't take my eyes off his beautiful, brown muscled frame. He pushed my hands down until I was touching his erection. I began stroking him. He started touching my neck and pulling me closer. I weakly attempted to pull away.

"Nooo, I can't," But I really wanted to.

" You can……no one will know except us." He whispered.

I had never done anything like this before.

Before I could think he kissed me and I kissed him back.

His lips were soft and wet

We kissed again, I moaned.

I was caught in the moment. I couldn't stop. Before I knew it, my head was going down below his waist. I was kissing and licking him. I didn't stop. I continued licking until he came in my mouth. He held my head tightly.

"Don't go," he said as I stood up.

I quietly and quickly walked into the bathroom and rinsed my mouth with the mouthwash that was sitting on the sink. I walked out of the bathroom. I looked at him and our eyes locked, neither of us said a word. I walked to the door, hand on the knob. I turned around for one last glance.

I couldn't go yet

I kicked off my shoes, pulled off my pants, pulled down my panties, and walked toward him.

His erection had returned.

I climbed onto the bed and slowly lowered myself on top of him. It felt so right. I didn't want to stop, so I didn't. I was on top of him until the end.

I climbed off of him.

I went into the bathroom and washed.

I wasn't sure how I felt.

I walked toward the door. I looked back at him. He was smiling. He blew me a kiss. I walked out and back to the nurses' station. The two CNAs were still asleep. I was a little bit ashamed, but then I thought .... I wasn't.

*** Sins of Nurses***

"Do not take life too seriously. You will never get out of it alive."

-Elbert Hubbard

Chapter 19

NO WAY

It usually takes about 2 hours to pass medications, and depending on where you work, this could take anywhere from the standard 2 hours to three or four hrs. I was working at this nursing home, where it usually took 3-4 hours to pass the medications. It took this long for several reasons.

One, you were responsible for about 30 residents.

Two, some were confused

Three, some were gone to do some form of therapy

Four, some might be participating in some kind of activity

Five, some were smokers and might be hanging out on the smoke patio, they would sit there for hours

Oh yeah, and you had several residents who had g-tubes.

All of these things made this particular assignment very

lengthy. We all hated it, we had complained to management about dividing assignments based on acuity. They had a meeting and said that the assignments would stay just as they were based on location.

There were three nurses on this floor with about 95 residents. We really should have had four nurses. But then, by now you know how things are in Nursing homes.

The facility wasn't about to spend any money for another nurse. They had already given us a treatment nurse. That helped a great deal but we still needed more help. One of the nurses went on vacation for a week and the facility hired an agency nurse to come in for that week. We normally rotate the assignment so that no one is stuck with the hard assignment every week. However, when the agency nurse came, we, of course, gave her the assignment that sucked. A typical practice. We explained to her that she should get started as early as possible because her assignment was difficult. She smiled and said ok. Around 8am, Betty, the other nurse working with me, got started with her med pass. Around 1030am, Betty and I returned to the nurses' station to see the agency nurse sitting there.

We laughed, "She is never going to get out of here today, she hasn't even started."

We know that whoever does that assignment won't return until about 1130am (if they are lucky).

Betty and I looked at each other, and I said to her jokingly, "If you don't get started, you are never going to get done?"

She responded matter of factly,

"I'm done, I finished a few minutes ago."

I almost spat out my coffee. Betty choked.

Then Betty asked her, "You're done with everything?"

"Yep!" She replied

Betty and I gave each other a look. We immediately speculated as to what kind of nurse she was. She was the kind who flushed medication down the toilet; nobody gets their medication kind of nurse.

Betty and I hurried down the hall; we could not wait to start gossiping and analyzing her.

"Look at her, sitting there smug as if she doesn't have a care in the world," Betty said.

"There is no way she could have possibly finished that assignment, that quickly," I said.

Then Betty said, "We've been here for years and, we KNOW the residents and can't finish that quickly. How can she come in here, not know the residents and finish in less than 2 hrs?"

NO FUCKING WAY!

She had to be throwing away her pills. Surely she must be flushing all of the medicine. We gossiped and speculated for quite a while until we realized that we were getting behind in our own work.

The next day another nurse came in from the agency, and we give her the same assignment. We gave her the same speech about getting started early. After this, we all headed out to pass our medications, and this was around 8am. Betty and I returned close to 1030am. The new nurse was nowhere to be found. 11am, and she still hadn't returned. She returned by 12pm and falls into the chair at the nurses' station.

"OH, MY GODDDDD, how do you guys get through this assignment, it's unreal?"

We explained to her that we know it was a tough assignment and that we rotate weekly to give each other a break from it. She was a good sport about it. She knew that we were taking a break from the assignment and dumping it on her at the same time. Our shift ended at 3:30pm, but I think she wasn't able to leave until well after 4pm, which is what one of the CNAs had said. The next day, which is Wednesday, the nurse from Monday had returned again. Same routine; we all left at 8am, Betty and I returned to the nurses' station around 1015am. We walked down the hall toward the nurses' station, laughing and talking about something someone had said. When we arrived there, she was sitting and doing her charting. She stated that she had finished a short time ago. "Wow," I said to her.

"We all hate that assignment because it takes so long to complete everything. How in the world do you finish so quickly?" She didn't answer.

Betty and I found time to gossip about it later. We continued to speculate.

Thursday came, she returned again.

This time Betty and I had a plan, we were going to watch her.

We start the same way as before. We all started out at 8am. I went down my hall, Betty down her hall, and the agency nurse went down her hall. Betty and I doubled back to watch her. We peered at her from down the hall. We saw her go into the cart and get medicine, pour a cup of water, go into the room, return empty handed, medicine gone. We observed her. She wasn't moving at any fast pace. She didn't appear to be a super nurse who was moving at some lightning speed. Betty and I gossiped again.

"She's giving out something; it must be a vitamin or something."

We figured she was too smart to simply not pass the pills. We thought that she just didn't give the particular medicines that were ordered. She gave a vitamin or something and kept it moving.

She only gave the medicines that she **had** to give.

We knew she had some difficult residents on that hall. We figured that if it were a difficult patient, she probably didn't even try to give medication. We watched her from down the hall.

We speculated that if the patient says, "No, I don't want it," she says, "okay, fine."

I mean, what else could she be doing? We asked each other. We were stumped. At one point, she looked down the hall and saw us talking and staring at her. She smiled at us. We smiled back. We kept speculating and gossiping. We were getting behind in **our own work** worrying about the agency nurse and how she got her work finished so early.

Betty and I both finished just after 10:30am that day. When we returned to the nurses' station, there she sat drinking coffee and reading the paper.

"Hey, you two, finally done with your med pass?" she said. NO WAY !!!

Sins of Nurses

"The ultimate tragedy is not the oppression and cruelty by the bad people but the silence over that by the good people." -Martin Luther King,Jr.

Chapter 20

THEY WANTED HER DEAD

As nurses, we don't always have control over the things that happen while we work. I guess some might disagree with the story that I am about to tell, but like all of the other stories. They are my stories, things that have happened to other Nurses as told to me, things that I have observed with my own eyes or things that I have experienced. Most importantly, they are my beliefs and opinions. And in my opinion, for whatever their reason, this family killed the mother.

There was a resident Mrs.Jakes. She was always climbing out of bed and, unfortunately, always falling. We always had to call the family for her. I think she had already fallen twice in the past week. She was a little bit confused, but overall she was in pretty good health.

So she falls for the third time this week, she hits her head this time. Her Nurse calls the Physician, who said to send her to the hospital to rule out any possible unseen head trauma. Off she went.

She returned from the hospital 3 days later, she was now my patient. She has a Foley catheter and has been placed on an NPO {nothing by mouth} status, which meant not to give her any food. So when I arrive and see the orders, I am a little confused as to why she is NPO.

What is the reason?

There is no swallow study in her chart. There were no orders for any evaluations of speech or swallowing.

There just didn't appear to be any reason for her NPO status. Nothing to support why she would not be allowed to eat other than the physicians order that she remain NPO.

"So are we to give her ice chips? I ask Sherry, the Unit Manager?"

"Let me call the doctor and clarify the orders."

"Ok, thanks, Sherry."

In the meantime, she is still doing what she usually does, trying to get out of bed and irritated that we won't give her any food.

She keeps repeating the same thing over and over.

"Why won't you give me food? I'm hungry!!" she says over and over.

The manager returns and says that she is to remain NPO and that she will be followed by Hospice.

"HOSPICE?" I exclaim.

"Why?" I ask the Unit Manager.

"Nurse Green, she's NPO, and she's Hospice, its what the family wants," Sherry says as she walks away.

Day 2 Her daughter in law appears. She is there for a few hours. Mrs. Jakes is still NPO. They say that a Hospice Nurse will be in later this evening. I didn't see her before I left at 3pm.

Mrs. Jakes is Hospice because that is what the family wants for her.

Day 3, Mrs. Jakes is quieter these days, no more complaining of being hungry.

Her Hospice Nurse arrives at the facility and sets the record straight for me.

"Why is she on hospice I ask her?"

She doesn't have any debilitating disease, no cancer, just some confusion, and a history of falling, I don't get it.

I'm asking the hospice nurse who wrote the order.

"Nurse Green, Mrs. Jakes, is under the care of Hospice, are we clear?"

I walk away from her and take my break. I'm pissed.

I return and find that she has now placed Mrs. Jakes on morphine if she needs it for pain.

What pain? This is Bullshit!

Day 4, no food or water, just ice chips for Mrs.Jakes

Mrs. Jakes is weak and not trying to get out of bed anymore. She is merely lying in bed, whispering that she is thirsty.

The daughter in law comes to the nurse's station and says that her mother in law is in pain, and needs morphine.

The nurses were all talking and speculating about the son and daughter in law and the way they kept requesting Morphine for Mrs. Jakes.

I knew that she had just gotten morphine about 2 hours ago.

I told her that I would come and assess Mrs. Jakes in a minute or two. She gave me a strange look.

I arrive at Mrs. Jakes room and observe.

She is lying quietly, she is not moaning, she doesn't appear to be any kind of distress or pain. Her eyes open as I stand there.

"Hi Mrs. Jakes, how are you feeling? Are you having pain right now sweetie?"

She replies "no, I'm just thirsty" "….ok, we'll get you some ice chips."

I tell her daughter in law, I think she's fine right now, she had something for pain a little while ago, and I'll monitor her. I know the dangers of giving morphine to a patient like this. I wasn't comfortable with what I thought was happening.

I again expressed my concerns regarding the requests for morphine from the daughter in law to my Director of Nursing, this time.

She said that I should document thoroughly.

I did so, I charted in her progress note what had transpired with the daughter in law requesting pain medication.

I hoped the other Nurses' were doing the same.

Two days later. I arrive for my shift and the night shift nurse who has verbalized and shared my same concerns. Immediately grabs me and pulls me into an empty room to talk. She says that the family has been in the facility all night and have been calling precisely every two hours demanding that she give Mrs.Jakes morphine around the clock.

"What are they trying to do, they are going to kill her!"

Is this their plan?

For whatever their reason, they don't want her around anymore. She's been here for years.

So the daughter in law arrives very early this morning.

The first thing that the daughter in law does is walk to Mrs. Jakes room and then comes to the Nurses station and says that her mother in law needs something for pain. I tell her the same thing that I've said every day for the past week,

"I'll come and check her in a minute or two"...

The daughter in law then says, "and when you come, bring the morphine."

I go to the resident's room without the morphine.

My assessment begins when I enter the room. I first observe her, she is not moaning, she appears asleep and to be calm. I check her heart rate and her breathing. Both are within normal limits and steady. There is nothing about her that gives me any indication that she is in pain. I try to arouse her, she doesn't easily arouse. Her eyes open, I ask her if she is hurting, she doesn't respond. Just staring at me, expressionless.

I tell the daughter in law " let's give it a little bit, I'll come back in about half an hour she appears to be comfor"….and before I finish my statement.

She starts yelling," what is your damned problem? Every time I ask you to give her something for the pain, you seem to have a problem with it!"

I explain to her that I am doing my job. I continue to tell her that when I assess her, and if I think for one second that she is in pain, I will give her something.

"You stay right here and you better not go anywhere, I'm calling my husband"…she's dialing a number.

I walk away…I'm halfway down the hall, and she yells for me to return……..I return.

She shoves her cell phone in my face and says that I need to speak to her husband. I take the phone.

"I don't know who you are, but you had better give my mother some goddamned morphine, and you'd better give it to her now."

"I'm on my way there, and you better have given her some morphine before I get there." I begin to explain ....click....he hangs up.

They call the hospice nurse themselves. The hospice nurse calls me 10 minutes later with an order from the physician to now give Mrs. Jakes morphine (at an increased dose) every 2 hours around the clock starting immediately.

Once an order comes from the physician there is nothing else, you can do.

I get the morphine and I go to the room to medicate Mrs. Jakes. She is not awake, she is making no sound, she appears to be sleeping soundly. She doesn't arise when I call her name and touch her. I take the dropper and give her an increased dose of morphine as is ordered. I put it in her mouth, under her tongue. About an hour later the son arrives, goes to the room speaks to his wife. He storms to the nursing station

"You're fucking lucky!" he says to me. He walks away

I don't say a word. I am fighting back my emotions, my thoughts and my personal opinion..

I give her the morphine every two hours during my 8-hour shift.

I was so upset. I went into the locked medication room and I started to cry. The nurse who was to relieve me arrived early. I guess she had searched for me, and someone told her that she could find me in the medication room.

She knocked on the medication room door, I opened it and tried to hide the fact that I had been crying.

I could hardly talk.

I managed to tell her everything that I was feeling. She began to cry. She offered to pray with me and told me not to worry because she was not going to worry, either. She said that we should know that whatever happens, "this is all between those people and God and that God knew our hearts, and that was enough."

"At the rate that we are medicating her, she's going to be dead by morning," I said.

We hugged each other.....I gave her report and left. When I arrived the next morning, the nurse came to me, she just stared and gave me a look....my heart sank....

"Mrs. Jakes died last night?"I asked.

She nodded, yes.

Sins of Nurses

"I'm not upset that you lied to me, I'm upset that from now on I can't believe you."

-Friedrich Nietzsche

Chapter 21

While they slept, they slept

I had just finished a night shift at this nursing home. It was the night from hell. I don't usually work night shifts, but I decided to do so for a short while, I needed the extra money. I was working through the agency again. I had three children at home…one in high school, one in middle school, and one in preschool. I was responsible for about 50 patients. I was pissed. I had gotten there at 11pm and had assessed that I had a shit load of work to do before I left at 7am. I immediately start "pulling my meds" so that I'm one step ahead and can leave on time in the morning. There were four nursing assistants on shift with me tonight. I had vaguely been introduced to them earlier. I walked up and down the three halls that I was responsible for, I was looking for everyone, the nursing assistants. I didn't see anyone. I finally found everyone, all four, propped in chairs with pillows and blankets asleep. I coughed and called to them and asked if anyone had done their rounds and checked their residents. They had only been there for about an hour, and there was no way they had done their work. They all grumbled that they had. I knew that they hadn't. I told them I would go down the hall and check, and if I found any resident who was wet or soiled, they would need to get up and check their people.

"You do that." one of them said sarcastically.

I know it might seem as if I was giving them an ok to do this, but I was not. You have to understand how things typically work with CNAs. Most nursing assistants have been doing what they have been doing for a very long time, and they know that they have management in their pockets.

I went down the hall and checked the rooms. Almost everyone I came across was wet and or soiled. I was irritated.

So fucking lazy! I thought to myself.

I was approaching one of the rooms at the end of the hall when I heard a faint cry for help. I walked into the room and did not see anyone. I turned around to leave and then I heard it again…"help!" It's coming from the bed by the window. I rushed over. The resident was wedged between the bed and the wall. I started yelling for help. No one came. I was at the north end of the hall, the CNAs were at the most south end from me, and they were all asleep. I did not want to hurt him, but he was too heavy for me to pull up. If I move the bed or he will crash to the floor.

I couldn't even push him. I had to leave him there and run for help.

I ran to the day room.

"I need help right away !! Who has Mr. Morrison in room 2112?" No one answered.

I yell it this time. "Who has the resident in room 2112? He's on the floor and I need some help!"

"You mean you can't do it yourself?" One of the CNAs commented.

"Seems like you have all the answers!" Another one said.

"If I don't get some help right now, I'm calling the director of nursing!"

I ran back down the hall.

I hear one of the nursing assistants behind me.

"I thought you were super nurse!" she said as she entered the room.

"I don't need to hear all of that; just help me get him back into bed," I said to her.

We got him back into the bed. I checked him over, he did not appear to have any injuries or bruises and his vital signs were normal.

Now I had an incident report to write on top of all the work I already have to do. Later on, I wrote out my incident report, along with four reports against the CNAs sleeping all night.

I was pretty sure nothing was going to happen to them.

It was now 4 am, and I started my morning waking up residents to give them medication.

Nobody wanted it. I could not rouse anyone.

The nursing assistants were getting everyone up and putting him or her in wheelchairs before 5am. As if, they had somewhere to go. The facilities policy (as with many of them) said that half of the residents must be out of bed before the arrival of the next shift.

I'm still attempting to perform my medication pass. It's difficult enough to give pills, but they all had these cans of supplement that they needed to drink.

On a good day, most of the residents' wouldn't' drink half of these health shakes. The dietician wanted us to get them to drink a can of this 2-3 times daily.

I tried in the first couple of rooms. I then just started to pour it out, I couldn't leave it on the cart and if you didn't give it to them, you would have to answer to management and the doctors.

None of whom could care less that its 4am and you can't get anyone to drink this stuff. Same with the pills, all the residents had pills and more pills. I tried to give them medicine but they did not want it and there was no coaxing at 4 in the morning. Nobody was getting anything. They won't drink and they won't take the pills. I was throwing away more than I was giving. I felt like screaming. At the same time, I was trying to check blood sugars as well. It was all absurd. Before I knew it, my relief arrived and only half of the medication had been given. I gathered it all and flushed it down the toilet.

All of it!!!

I then charted in the MAR that I had given it. I ran out of that hellhole. I never went back. The office called me a few days later and said that the facilities director wanted to speak to me regarding the reports that I had written against the nursing assistants. I called from the office. They asked me if I was sure that things happened the way that I had written them as happening. I assured her that it was correct. She then told me that the four nursing assistants had written statements as well and had charged that I slept at the desk all night and did no work. They had to wake ME up every time they needed assistance. They had said that the reason that I wrote disciplinary reports against them was because I knew that they were going to write a report against me.

I held the phone, I was silent. No need to defend myself. She then asked me what I had to say about their statements. I simply stated that there was no truth to their statements. She thanked me and ended the phone call.

I never heard anything else. My understanding from friends that had gone there after me was that nothing had changed and that the four nursing assistants were still there.

I heard that they had done an investigation and found that "I" was not truthful and that I wasn't welcome back to their facility. And that was that. It usually ended that way.

Sins of Nurses

"Be yourself; everyone else is already taken."

-Oscar Wilde

Chapter 22

DAD, PUT SOME PANTS ON

Mr. White arrived at our facility at about 10:45am on a Thursday morning. He was an 82-year-old African American gentleman that stood about 5′6″ in height and weighed about 160 lbs. He was accompanied by his daughter Angel. I was sitting at the nurses' station when they came through the door of the unit. I knew I was getting an admission, so I was expecting them. I introduced myself and walked the two back to his private room, they were adamant that he have a private room, and they paid to secure him one. Angel's husband was there, he had brought in a few boxes and some items of clothing. I told them to excuse me while I walked back to the nurses' station to order his lunch and to get his paperwork. When I returned,

I heard the daughter say, "Daddy, why don't you put your pants back on while the nurse is talking to you and finishing with the paperwork?" He replied that he didn't need to put on any pants, that he didn't have anything to hide, and that I had probably seen it all before.

I laughed to myself

The daughter turned to me and asked if I wanted her father to put on pants. I replied that he was okay; after all, I could see that he had on boxers, a long dress shirt, and thermal underwear.

"If he doesn't want to put on pants, that's fine," I say.

As the morning went on, it seemed as though she was becoming more and more irritated and annoyed that her father wouldn't put his pants on. Her husband was laughing at his wife's annoyance.

She gave him the…not a damn thing is funny look.

I gave them some privacy to get things settled, I return about 30 mins later to ask a few more questions of Mr. White, who was standing and fidgeting in the closet.

I asked him if he would have a seat so that I could go over a few things.

"We can discuss your health, your medications and then I have a few forms for you to sign." He seemed to be deliberately ignoring me. He continued to fold his clothes and to unpack his boxes. He was there for rehab and strength training. He probably wouldn't be at our facility for more than a few weeks. His daughter began to plead with him, "Daddy, please put your pants on until 'I' leave!" He started singing. "I'mmmm nottt puttttinnnggg on anythinnngggg and you'rrreee goonnna be okkkkkk."

"I can't do this," she exclaimed.

She was even starting to annoy ME.

It was no big deal, gosh, I thought.

I see residents in their underwear all the time. Her husband then said to her, "Why don't you wait downstairs while he's talking to the nurse?" She didn't say a word; she turned and walked out of the room. Mr. White then turned around. My mouth fell open. Although it was, clear that Mr. White had on boxers and thermals it became immediately clear as to why the daughter wanted him to put pants on. Mr. White had been greatly blessed.

You couldn't help but notice that he had a huge penis, a very long penis that was so big that it bulged through his boxers and thermals. There was no ignoring it. I tried not to stare. He came dancing toward me. "See something you like?" He asked me while gyrating his hips. I had to put on my Grammy winning face.

"Mr. White! Sir, please have a seat while we go over these forms."

He maintained a huge grin on his face. He sat down into the chair in front of me. He sat the way almost any 70 something-year-old man would sit. Legs wide open. Not that I was looking, but it looked as though his penis was sitting in the chair by itself. I was trying to stay focused. I didn't want to smile.

I didn't want to seem nervous, either.

His son-in-law said to him, "Pops please cover yourself up man!"

He refused and responded, "Why do I have to cover anything up, we're all adults here."

The son-in-law began to laugh and shake his head; he shrugged his shoulders at me as if to say, "The ball is in your court."

I started asking my questions.

Mr. White answered me appropriately, only occasionally winking his eye at me.

I think that he even licked his lips once or twice.

What were we in for?

I finished asking all of my questions and he signed my forms. There, admission complete! I thanked him, gathered all of my paperwork and left the room. I walked down the hall to the nurses' station and sat down. One of the CNAs walked by.

"Nurse, why is your face so red?" I started laughing.

"You don't want to know." She sat down next to me and said. "I know this is going to be good, why are you so red?" I tell her. She laughed something terrible.

I'm going to go and see for myself! "She says.

" Then, he is now your patient!" I tell her.

"So, you go right ahead."

She heads down the hall to his room. She comes back about 10 minutes later. She is shaking her head.

"You don't want to know," she says.

"You don't want to know." We start to laugh.

Sins of Nurses

"Don't cry because it's over, smile because it happened."

-Dr. Seuss

Chapter 23

TOO MUCH TV?

There are so many things that happen in a nursing home, some things are good, some are bad, and some are funny. The work is so hard, and some days you have to laugh to keep from crying. I'm working another double shift 7-3pm and 3pm-1130pm. It's going to be a long day, and I'm already having a really rough day. I'm fighting with Mr. Beasley to take his medicine. Trying to reason with him. He usually watches television all day. The CNAs have him watching music videos. Whenever I go into a resident's room, and I find that their television is on one of the popular music videos or reality TV shows, I always change the channel to something more appropriate. I didn't do that with Mr. Beasley because he liked all of the half-naked women dancing in the videos. I turn down the volume on the TV and stand in front of it. "Mr. Beasley, I will leave your room after you take your medicine." He starts singing a song. "Drop down and get your eagle on girl, drop down and get your eagle on girlllllllllllllll." He keeps singing loudly.

"Mr. Beasley, please!!" He stops for a minute.

"What?" he says.

"Will you please take this medicine?"

"Are you going to go away if I take it?"

"Yes, I am, and I won't bother you anymore on my shift."

"Well, okay," he says and throws them in his mouth, chewing them ferociously.

"Take it down to the floor, drop down, and…."

I turn the volume back up on the TV and head toward the door. Just as I reach it, I see Mr. Jordan running by without his shoes on.

"Mr. Jordan, go back to your room and get your shoes, you know you could fall without them!"

He does a U-turn and heads back to his room. I push my cart a few feet over and begin to prepare the medications for the resident in the next room, Mrs. Morrison. I get all of the medicine together. I have a cup of crushed pills with applesauce.

Someone tell me how you crush fish oil? Better yet try getting a resident to take it once you've squeezed out the contents and added them to a mixture of pills and applesauce.

Nevermind, I snip the tips and pour the stinky, sticky contents into a cup.

A cup of liquid Colace.

A cup of liquid Multivitamin.

A measured syringe of 5cc Dilantin.

A cup of water.

A cup of her nutritional supplement.

I lock the cart, and then I hear this weird clicking and shuffling sound. I turn around, and there is Mr. Jordan again. He is running toward me. I yell for him to stop and slow down before he falls and hurts himself.

"Okay, nurse," he says.

I look down at his shoes, and I notice that he has on two pair!

"What the hell," I think to myself.

I then stand in front of him so that he can't move.

"Mr. Jordan, why do you have on two pairs of shoes, I mean how did you get two pairs of shoes on?" I exclaim.

He just stares at me.

One pair is clearly bigger than the other.

He's "borrowed" someone else's shoes.

Mr. Jordan is known for borrowing things that don't belong to him

I look closer. He has on two pair of pants and three shirts and a coat. It's probably 80 degrees outdoors. I grab ahold of his hand and start to walk him back to his room. Then I remember all of my medicine.

"Oh shit!"

I let go of his hand and tell him," wait right here and don't move. I'll be right back."

I turn and head towards my cart, grab all of the medicine, put it inside the carts top drawer, and then lock it.

I turn around and look .....Mr. Jordans' gone.

I don't see him anywhere.

No Worries, I know I will see him again.

Mr. Beasley stands in the doorway of his room.

"Drop down......," he sings.

"Mr. Beasley!" I yell to him.

"Go back into your room, I don't want to hear that rap song anymore!"

He gives me the finger and slams the door to his room.

Usually, whenever you find all residents, singing a particular song, it's because it's what is popular on the television, and the CNAs are usually putting the residents' TVs on these channels while they are working with a resident in their room.

Some of the CNAs will even teach residents the lastest songs.

It can be funny sometimes. Most of the time, it's just annoying.

I shake my head, and I return to the cart to get my medicines. As I take everything out, I notice that my applesauce has begun to liquefy.

"Shit," I think to myself.

I gather it anyway without getting new pills. My cup of liquid applesauce, my cup of Colace, my cup of the multivitamin, my syringe of Dilantin, a cup of water, and a cup of nutritional supplement. I knock and head inside Mrs. Morrison's room. She is sitting there and waiting for me.

“Good morning Mrs. Morrison, I have your medication.” She is lying in her bed, and it’s totally flat.

I need the head of her bed up if I’m going to give her medicine while she is still in it.

She is humming to herself softly.

Mrs. Morrison, could you sit up for me, please? She doesn’t move, so I decide to just let the bed up and give her the medicine there.

Where is the bed controller? No controller. CRANKS!

Are you kidding me?

I do not have time for these old ass beds! I bend over and wayyyyyyyy down; Crank out, attempting to turn, ... it's like turning an old rusted handle.

I’m bent over, back hurting, rusty crank handle barely turning, head eventually up.

She barely looks my way, but she is at least sitting up. She continues to hum to herself.

I sit all of the medicine down in front of her and take a seat because I know this is going to take a while. Anything you give to her, she takes her time in swallowing it. This is just the way she is, and that is the way it goes sometimes.

I know that I’m going to be here for a while.

I might as well start watching the videos myself because she is going to take 5 or 6 minutes before she is done.

"Mrs. Morrison, here you go, take your medicine." I raise the spoon to her mouth to get her started. She opens her mouth wide, and just as I put the spoon close to her mouth, she purses her lips and kisses the spoon.

"Mrs. Morrison open your mouth, please, nice and wide for me," I say.

She then opens her mouth nice and wide. As soon as I place the spoon close to her lips, she purses her lips closed as if I were giving her a lemon.

She leans forward and then nibbles the smallest amount humanly possible from the spoon.

I talk to her for a minute before trying again.

"Here you go, Mrs. Morrison open wide." I put the spoon near her mouth again.

This time instead of pursing her lips for the tiniest amount, she licks the medicine on the tip of the spoon.

"opennn opennn opennn" She closes her mouth.

I'm about ready to throw all of this medicine into the toilet. I give her a sip of water, which she takes. I then give her sips of her nutritional supplement. She is drinking this today.

I pour drops of each liquid onto the spoon. She continues to purse her lips and take the tiniest taste of each. I try the crushed pills again. As soon as she opens her mouth wide, I hurriedly dump a huge spoonful into her mouth. I immediately try to give her the supplement to drink and get it down.

She turns her head away from the supplement and starts to just spit out the medicine. She

spitting it on the floor. It runs out of her mouth and unto her clothing. I just stare at her. I shake my head.

I go into the bathroom, grab a towel, return and wipe her mouth and clothing. I flush everything that is left down the toilet.

"hmmm...hmmm," she is humming as I walk out of the door.

I go to my cart to get medicine for my next resident. I hear the clicking and shuffling again. I turn, and it's Mr. Jordan. He still has on layers of clothing and two pair of shoes. I grab his arm as he shuffles by. I begin to walk him to his room. I look around; I don't see any nursing assistants. I get to his room, I sit him down on the bed, and help him to take off some of his clothing.

I take off one pair of the two pair of his shoes. I place them in his closet. Two shirts off and a pair of pants later. I tell myself to remember to have a nursing assistant grab the bigger shoes and find out whom they belong to. I walk down the hall to my cart and begin to "pull" pills again. I am crushing the next set of pills. It's Depakote. It shouldn't be crushed but the facility is too cheap to buy a liquid version. I continue to crush it.

I think out loud, "5cc multivitamin, 20cc potassium…."

I hear clicking and shuffling.

It's Mr. Jordan running past me again, and he has the two pair of shoes on again.

"Mr. Jordan!" I yell to him. He keeps running. I yell behind him,

"You're going to fall, stop running and come here!" He turns the corner and runs into Mr. Givens. They both bump and fall to the floor. I run toward them, they appear to be uninjured. They both begin to laugh. Mr. Beasley appears in the doorway of his room. "Drop down and get your eagle on girl, drop down and get your eagle on…."

"Mr. Beasley, go back into your room with all of that singing!" I yell to him.

He slams his door shut. I help Mr. Jordan and Mr. Givens to chairs. They are both now looking confused. A small knot is starting to form on the head of Mr. Givens. All I am thinking is that I haven't finished passing medications; now, I have to get vital signs, call doctors, and everything that goes along with filling out an incident report. Two incident reports.

I leave them sitting at the nurses' station, and I tell them both not to move and to wait for me.

"Don't either of you get out of these chairs, I'll be right back."

I leave and go to get my cart hoping that I will see a CNA who can help me. I don't see anyone in sight. I grab my cart and head back down the hall to where they are sitting. They are both gone. I look around.

"Shit!!"

I'll have to find them later. I continue my med pass.

Sins of Nurses

"Forgiveness is not an occasional act, it is a constant attitude." -ML King, Jr.

Chapter 24

SABOTAGE

I have always considered myself a person who hated no one. Hate is a useless emotion that I choose not to give life to. Yet, in all of my years in nursing. In all of the places that I have worked; (at the writing of this book, there was only one now, there are quite a few)one particular CNA makes me use this word. I hated that certified nursing assistant, that woman. I hated her with everything inside of me. I couldn't begin to tell all of the things that she did to me, but I'll try to mention the most memorable ones. I think the thing that first brought Jocelyn to my attention when I started that job was that she always left the unit. She would leave for long periods of time, and no one knew where she actually was. The other nursing assistants would cover for her. I remember being frequently irritated regarding never being able to find her. I tried everything to try and keep track of her disappearing acts, nothing seemed to work. I found that I was always looking for her and not finding her. It seems like locating her should have been simple seeing the way that she looked. She probably stood around 5'9-5'10' and weighed well over 200lbs.

To make matters worse, she was ugly (inside and out), unprofessional, loud, brash, and ghetto in every sense of the word. She wore outlandish colorful wigs unbecoming of her, and she was built like a dump trunk. Everything about her spoke, "trashy."

Jocelyn would pull these disappearing acts; one minute, she was on the floor, and then the next, she was gone.

I had to do something. I finally came up with something that I thought might work.

I implemented a system of signing in and out of the unit whenever you left the floor. Some of the cna's complained as they knew that this signing in and out was really meant to target Jocelyn. They thought that it wasn't fair and it wasn't. But if you know cna's, then you know they were all doing their fair share of missing acts from the floor. But, Of course, Jocelyn didn't like it. She knew that It was aimed at tracking her.

This was when she decided that she "really" did not like me.

Whenever she walked by me, she would give me a smirk.

I was causing her to have to work.

Our unit manager, Willy, was afraid of her, and everyone knew it. He wouldn't say anything to her unless he was backed into a corner and had to. She was the worst CNA in the building, and I think she got the first write up in her little career from me for her multitude of resident infractions.

Over the next few weeks, we had run-in after run-in. I would check her work, I would check her patients. Most of the time, as I knew they would be, they were unattended to and appeared to have not been turned (the protocol was that they be turned every 2 hours to prevent skin breakdown and bed sores). She was awful, and I found most of the time, her patients to be soaking wet, have crusted feces, generally uncared for.

These things contributed to my general dislike for Jocelyn.

I was working one evening shift. Making my rounds and checking the residents on my halls. I went into the room of a resident with whom Jocelyn was the caregiver. I checked the resident, Mrs. Gray, and found that she was soaked in urine and feces.

I left the room to get Jocelyn.

As usual, Jocelyn was missing, she hadn't signed out, and No one seemed to know where she was.

I searched the halls, she wasn't anywhere.

Eventually, I saw her getting off the elevator, returning to the floor. I reminded her that she should be signing out whenever she leaves the floor. I told her that her residents needed to be attended to…etc…etc… She became irate and loud and stated that I was picking on her and that she was going to report me.

"In the meantime (I told her), please go and take care of Mrs. Gray."

She stormed into the room of Mrs. Gray. I could hear her mumbling what I was sure were insults about me. I didn't care. I wanted her to do the work that she was paid to do.

I was sitting at the nurses' station talking to the other nurse when Jocelyn stormed back out to the desk a few minutes later yelling

" that resident is not wet !"

"you have a problem, you're picking on me!"

I looked at her and then I looked away. This time, I had the smirk. I knew she was telling a lie.

Because I knew that Jocelyn was going to deny that here residents were uncared for, I had asked Sandra the other Nurse that I was working with if she wouldn't mind verifying the condition of Mrs. Gray. She didn't really want to as she knew that it was Jocelyns' patient, and like everyone else, she was afraid of Jocelyn.

No one wanted to be on Jocelyn's bad side.

It was rumored that she had done things to other nurses' cars in the past.

The rumor was that she had once slashed a nurse's tires.

That she poured sugar down the gas tank of another nurse.

She had also threatened multiple nurses with physical harm.

None of these things were of any significance to me as I had grown up on the south side of Chicago in public housing.

After going into the room and checking Mrs. Gray just to verify that she was uncared for Sandra returned to the Nurses station and sat down next to me.

Once Jocelyn stormed away, Sandra exclaimed

"She's crazy, that resident is unclean and wet, and she hasn't done anything."

I looked at her, "Exactly."

"This is what I go through every time I work with her," I said to Sandra.

Without having taken care of Mrs. Gray, Jocelyn walking into the resident TV room and simply sat there staring at me.

I called her name, she ignored me.

I didn't say another word to her but paged the facility supervisor to my floor.

Jocelyn jumped up and went to the room of Mrs. Gray.

When the supervisor arrived, I told her of what had happened, and the other nurse was my witness to this.

By this time, Jocelyn had come out of Mrs. Gray's room and began her loud and ignorant complaints that I was picking on her and that she had done her job. I looked at her and shook my head. The supervisor made a note of what I had said.

Nothing happened.

This is what is typical regarding CNA complaints by a Nurse.

NOTHING HAPPENS!!

It is the reason nurses have stopped complaining.

It doesn't matter.

The war between Jocelyn and myself became escalated after that.

Our next encounter….I was passing medication to residents who were sitting at the nurses' station. There were two residents sitting there. I knew them both well and had prepared their medicine. Legally, we are supposed to prepare the medicine of only one resident at a time.

Nevertheless, we bend the rules at times to get things done, especially if no one else is around; *and there was no one else around.*

I have my two prepared cups of medicine. I sit one cup of pills on my cart, and I walk a foot or two to one resident, and I give her medication with water. This only took a minute.

No other residents had come to the area, and no one seemed to be around.

When I turned around, the pills, which I had left on top of the cart, were gone.

Am I going crazy? I thought to myself.

There was no one else in sight. No one.

I was cautious that no resident was even close when I sat them there.

Jocelyn has me losing my mind !

I KNEW that I had prepared the medication, at least I thought so.

This is going to be a long day and I'm going crazy.

I prepared more medication and gave it to the other resident who was sitting there and patiently waiting.

I was still puzzled by the incident.

About 30 minutes later. Another CNA who was very quiet and who rarely said much, Salley came up to me and whispered,

"Can I talk to you for a minute?"

"Sure," I said

She wanted me to follow her into one of the empty resident rooms.

Once there, she closed the door and began, "You know that I keep to myself and that I don't like trouble, so please don't say anything…but I found these pills in the room sitting in front of Mr. Smith, and he was about to take them!"

I was trying to take in what she was saying.

She went on further to say that she had watched Jocelyn take the cup of pills from atop my cart while my back was turned.

She said that she wondered what she was going to do with them, so she followed her and noticed that she had gone into the room of Mr. Smith and had put them in front of him with a cup of water and walked away. She then stated that Jocelyn had left the floor telling one of the other CNA that she was going downstairs to report me to the Director of Nursing.

"She is probably going to try and get you fired, I'm not sure." She says as she shook her head.

She finished by saying that she grabbed the pills and brought them to me.

I was in shock.

I looked at the pills, they were the ones from earlier, they were indeed my pills.

I gave Salley a hug and thanked her.

She walked out of the room first.

I then walked out, in one direction and Salley in the other.

I went back to the nurses' station and sat there. I had just disposed of the pills when Jocelyn and the Director of Nursing stepped off the elevator.

Neither looked my way; they simply walked down the hall to the room where Jocelyn knew that she had left the pills.

They returned a short time later.

I noticed them, but I didn't look up, I kept to my charting.

A short time later, The Director called to the unit and asked me to come down to her office.

I walked in, closed the door, and sat down. There she proceeded to caution me regarding leaving medicine in the resident rooms at their bedsides.

I assured her that this was never a practice of mine and that I wasn't sure as to where this even came from. She then told me that "some" of the nursing assistants had noticed that I would leave pills in the residents' rooms and walk out.

I simply stared at her.

I denied this.

I felt that she knew what was happening.

There were no "some" nursing assistants, there was just one.

I told her that I would continue to practice nursing to the best of my ability and would be very careful in following the protocol of medicating one resident at a time and not turning my back on my medicine. I then told her of what Jocelyn had done. She advised me to speak to my unit manager regarding the incident and to let him handle things. The next day I wrote a statement charging that Jocelyn had purposely taken the medicine and sat it in front of a resident.

My need to try to punish Jocelyn was higher than the trouble I would get into for turning my back on my pills.

In the end, they simply spoke to her, and she denied it. After all, no one had seen her do this.

Nothing was done.

In another instance, there was a resident who I knew to be afraid of Jocelyn. You could just see her fear whenever Jocelyn was around. This was ignored because this resident was confused most of the time. Confused or not, she was afraid of Jocelyn.

I was giving me her medication when Jocelyn walked into the room one day. I could see the fear come across her face.

I asked her if she was ok.

"she hits me." The resident said.

I didn't let her say anymore, I went to grab a witness.

I grabbed Willy, the unit manager. He listened.

The resident repeated the same story regarding Jocelyn hitting her. We wrote everything in an incident report. To my surprise, they sent Jocelyn home pending an investigation. The resident's daughter came to the facility the next day. The resident told her daughter the exact story that she had told the supervisor and me. The daughter was pissed. They assured her that an investigation was being pursued regarding the incident. In the end, the findings were that they found the resident to be too confused and not credible enough to make such an accusation. They brought Jocelyn back two days later. During her time away from the facility, management had decided that it was best that Jocelyn and I no longer work on the same floor.

They put her on another floor. I didn't see her for a few weeks.

The next time that I saw her, I was sitting in the employee lounge. She sat close enough to me so that I could hear her. She spent the next few minutes going on and on "I will fuck up a nurse, I don't care about this job, I can get another one"!

"I will slap the shit out of her and keep walking, and it wouldn't be the first time," she went on to say as I listened. Eventually, I tired of listening to her threats and left the area.

Everyone warned me to stay away from her and to watch my back, and I did.

Eventually, this all fizzled down.

Soon the unit manager was fired, and an old supervisor returned.

Jocelyn wanted to return to my floor.

Jocelyn convinced this supervisor that there was simply a misunderstanding between us. This new supervisor went to bat to get her returned to the floor. It worked. She was allowed to come back to the floor to my dismay and against my protests. Once she returned, she started up again with her sneaky behavior. This time she had someone backing her up. Later and as it would happen to be, this supervisor was a lesbian.

(Don't worry, I'm going somewhere with this point.) She called me into her office one day. I went to her office and there sat Jocelyn. She had been crying. The supervisor asks her to repeat her story. She goes on to tell a story of overhearing me speaking to another nursing assistant and stating

" I don't like gay people."

"I don't think lesbian or gay people should be working with the elderly."

She went on further to say that she was personally offended, as she was gay and that I knew it (which I did not.)

I was shocked. Mouth open. I hadn't heard such a stupid story/lie in my life!

Was she really trying this? I didn't know if I wanted to laugh or cry.

There wasn't an ounce of truth in any of this, but it didn't matter. She had said it, and the new supervisor wasn't going to forget it any time soon.

I was pissed at the end of this conversation.

Of course, this supervisor didn't like me now.

This is all I need!

Shortly, thereafter I started to hear that this supervisor was making negative comments about me. I heard she was saying things like

"I behaved as if I was better than the other nurses ."

" That I thought that I was perfect."

"That I had a bad attitude."

I knew where all of this was going. I would probably be looking for another job if it were up to the two of them. The only problem is that I was a hardworking nurse, so finding a reason to fire me was a challenge. About a week later, I received a write up (reprimand) for something stupid. Something like I was difficult to work with and that she had many complaints regarding my attitude.

Eventually, she couldn't be bothered with the task of looking for a reason to fire me.

I guess one day, she just said, "Fuck it."

One minute I was working and passing medications, and the next minute, I was asked to go downstairs to the office of the Director of Nursing. I arrived, and there was the Director of nursing and my supervisor. My supervisor started by saying that I was difficult to get along with and that the nursing assistants thought that I was very unapproachable.

I listened.

The Director of Nursing then stated that someone had noted that I was "eating" and passing medications and that this was a violation of the facility infection control policy.

I stared at them, I continued to listen intensely.

I was fired on the spot.

They walked me back to the unit to get my things. They then walked me out of the building. I was hurt and devastated. I worked very hard and didn't deserve that.

I called one of my girl pals who I knew wasn't working that day. We met at a local Bar and Grill.

I ordered a drink. It was 11am. The server asked what we were celebrating. I told her that I had just been fired from my job. She smiled and said that I should expect a better position to come along. I had a margarita. They made it a double and gave it to me on the house. It only confirmed to me that working hard and doing the right thing in nursing would never be enough. I filed for unemployment. I figured I might as well take a month off for my inconvenience. It was denied. I appealed it. They scheduled a hearing. The finding was in my favor, and the report stated that I was found to be a credible candidate and that my previous employer was not. I won my case. I stayed home for a month, writing parts of this book.

Word of caution, and please know this. If one CNA or multiple CNAs don't like you, you might want to quit! I'm cut from a different type of cloth, very strong material, and I don't scare easily. But please, nurses weigh the risk that you take; you don't want to lose your license over bullshit!

Sins of Nurses

"I loved the thought of becoming a nurse until I became one."

-R.L Green

Chapter 25

PROMISES TO KEEP

Some facilities will do anything to keep their census up. This particular nursing home was one such place. It was no secret that the marketing team would go out in the evenings and canvas the streets to gather homeless and even drug-addicted men and women. Promise them a bed, food, clothing, and even drugs, excuse me, narcotics. Yes, narcotics. The homeless and drug addict saw a light in this. It all looked fantastic to them, more than they could ever hope for. The one thing that they didn't tell these people before getting them into the facility is that they couldn't come and go as they pleased. This was to change; they were going to work around that for the sake of numbers and dollars. I could write and will write many stories about this particular facility, its residents, and the things that happened there.

This story involves a drug-addicted middle-aged boyfriend and his equally drugged, addicted girlfriend.

They came into the facility looking scraggly, unclean, and psychotic. She had sores all over her body, and he had the same. He had one leg and was in a wheelchair. His amputated leg had a severe infection at the stump.

It would appear that if you are homeless, you don't care much about doctors' visits, even if your leg is about to fall off.

It turned out that he had a MRSA infection. He was to start a treatment of IV antibiotics and a few other much-needed medications.

We needed to get him started on IV antibiotics right away. It was just what we nurses wanted, a crack head with an IV access port and to fully gown, mask, and glove up every time you went into his room.

It gets worse!

He treated the nurses and cna's like trash, he talked to us very disrespectfully ordering us around and yelling if you didn't move quickly enough.

His girlfriend was in the room next door. She behaved the same. The two of them drove the staff crazy.

Management decided that a room change was needed, separating the two of them was in order.

They put him on the first floor and his girlfriend on the third floor. Every day she would come down and spend the day with him.

Guess what they did when they were alone?

Once behind closed doors, they would prop things against it to keep the staff out. We knew they were having sex.

We were told that it was their right to have sex! Even if it made all the staff uncomfortable.

We never actually caught them in the act, and no one wanted to.

If they weren't camping out in their rooms having sex, they were hanging around the nurses' station on each floor, begging for pain medication.

She would cry to any nurse who would listen to her to have all of these pains throughout her body.

She drove us crazy.

We knew it was a game. She was just seeking drugs.

Eventually, she got her way, and they put her on a narcotic pain medication every 4 hours, and every 4 hours like clockwork, she'd come to the nurses' station claiming that she was in severe pain and needed her medicine.

It was super irritating to us all.

We were professionals, not addiction counselors; most of us resented that we had to deal with these types of people.

The facility may have had 25-30 such people like these two.

It was crazy!!

They were even allowed to drink alcohol in their rooms.

This was a right reserved for only a select few, supposedly. There were a few 70-80-year-olds who were allowed to have an occasional glass of wine or beer. Management and the physicians had okayed this. I thought it was a nice idea. *Hell, when I'm 80 and sitting in a nursing home, I hope that I can have a nightly glass of wine to keep me sane.*

However, these newcomers were drug addicts!!

Who does this?

Sure, we had all heard of facilities doing this before but never to this degree.

Many of these people would leave out of the building to smoke marijuana and to do drugs.

Management was fully aware of this.

I guess you are wondering why none of us quit.

We needed our jobs, and as nursing home pay rates go, they paid a pretty decent rate, so we all stayed and dealt with it. Here we were, coming into work daily and having to deal with crackhead 1 and crackhead 2 as we called them behind their backs.

Crackhead 1 belonged on my floor, crackhead 2 wouldn't leave my floor unless she was going upstairs to get her legal drugs.

UUUUggghhh, they both grossed everyone out.

Management decided to move crackhead 1 into the room next to the nurses' station.

The premise was that they could monitor if not, control him better by moving him to a room near the nurses' station where the nurses could keep an eye on him. *A premise* Guess how that went? We watched him better, all right.

Anyway, whenever that door would open, the smell that would ooze from within was enough to make you gag. Sexual activity, infections, and no baths make for absolute repulsion anywhere near the nurses' station.

All of the nurses were complaining. It didn't do any good. The only thing that mattered was the census. The number of residents in that building who created paychecks for the owners. The reality was that our numbers were borderline, and we couldn't afford to lose any bodies.

Crackhead 1 would come to the nurses' station every 3 ½ hours and begin to ask for his pain medication. He would be redirected and told that he needed to wait 30 more minutes. He would literally sit at the nurses' station and stare at you for those 30 minutes. He was a scary-looking character but not one whom I was afraid of. He sat and stared to intimidate you. He would watch the clock and then when the time came to give him the narcotic, and you didn't get right up he would ACT A FOOL

I heard that the girlfriend did the same thing on the third floor.

As if that wasn't bad enough, they both continued to sneak out of the facility. The staff would be looking for them for hours, we'd give up and then they would show up saying that they had been sitting in the back of the building in the garden.

This was untrue.

Most of the nurses were starting to become fearful for their licenses dealing with all of the drug-addicted individuals in the building.

It was an endless cycle of them getting drugs in some form or another legally from the doctors at the facility via the nurses. Then disappearing from the facility for hours on end returning drunk or high and asking for the legal narcotics that we had for them.

This was also proving to be unsafe for the elderly who we were supposed to be protecting and caring for. These street persons were beginning to manipulate the other residents. Conning them out of money, clothes, whatever they could. We were concerned about this.

Management didn't seem to care. They were only concerned about the money being made from having beds filled.

It was a mess!

I have to start looking for another job.

I knew I couldn't continue to do this. These people were going to hurt someone.

One day after being outside of the building and returning under the influence, crackhead 1 came to the nurses' cart drunk and high, asking for his narcotics. I looked at him straight in his eyes and told him I wasn't giving him anything.

He started to curse me and to tell me all the things that he was going to do to me if I didn't get him his pain pills. I looked at him straight on and repeated myself

"I'm not giving you a thing." Then he began to threaten me.

"You don't want to play this again, nursie, get those pills. I know that I can have them." He yelled at me.

I looked at him and responded, "I'm not giving you shit!" This made him laugh. With a smirk on his face, he rolled away in his wheelchair. I should have known that that wouldn't be the end. He returned a short time later with my supervisor.

"Now, tell her what you said to me." He said.

I hesitated a little and then stated, "I'm not giving you any narcotics."

My supervisor then asked me if he were within the period to give him the narcotics? I replied that he was. She then asked,

"Then what is your reason for not giving them to him?"

It was obvious that he was under the influence of something; clearly, she was blind.

I asked her to step inside the nurses' station so that I could speak to her in private.

"He has been gone from the facility, he is high off of something, and he also appears under the influence of alcohol, and I don't feel comfortable giving him anything."

I further told her that I had charted all of this in his chart. She replied that if it were in the period in which he could have his pain medication, then she expected me to give him medication. I went to the narcotic box, took out the medicine, signed it out, and then went to where she sat waiting and set the pills down in front of her and asked her if she wouldn't mind giving him the narcotics. She looked over at him, just as his head began a slight nod. You could smell the alcohol from where he sat. She looked a bit startled and asked me why I would expect her to give him medication. I told her that I didn't feel comfortable giving him the pain medication, and since she was comfortable with the idea, could she please give them to him. She was taken aback. She snapped at me, "I don't have time to play this game with you just give him the pills!"

I looked at her and continued to stand my ground. I repeated my previous statement that if she felt so comfortable with giving him narcotics, she could give them to him herself and that I would chart that she had given him the medication.

I wasn't going to give him anything.

Why wouldn't she want to give medication to him?

After all, she was a registered nurse, and she had the pills sitting right in front of her with a cup of water. All she had to do was hand them to him.

She jumped up and turned to me, and just as she did so, crackhead 1 snatched the cup of pills from the countertop and swallowed them.

"Fuck yall!" He said as he wheeled away.

I looked at her, "I'll just document that you gave him his pills."

She stared at me as if she wanted to kill me.

"I'm writing you up." She stated.

"That's fine, I quit. Would you like me to leave now or finish my shift?"

She stared at me, "Finish your shift, please."

"No problem. " I replied.

This was an evening shift, so I got all of the 9pm nighttime medications ready. I started at 8pm, like always. Tonight I started with resident crackhead. He was high out of his head when I entered the room. He took all the pills that I gave to him in one gulp.

He winked his eye at me.

I winked my eye at him right back and walked out of the room.

I had given him 3 bisacodyls with his medication. I finished my shift. I then turned in my keys and my badge. I didn't return. (New nurses, remember that the choice is always yours. Be wise where you can.)

*** Sins of Nurses***

"A man is never more truthful than when he acknowledges himself a liar."

-Mark Twain

Chapter 26

FEEDING TIME

Most nurses and CNAs dislike it when it is time to feed residents. Nurses don't like it because it cuts into our time. We are already squeezing much into our 8 hr. day and feeding someone remains low on the list of priorities. CNAs have the same kind of sentiment. It's just too time-consuming.

Usually, the only staff members that don't mind feeding residents are the restorative aides (because they have to) and the staff who like to eat the residents' food.

Yessss, you actually have some staff persons that will eat directly from the residents' plates.

Others will get a tray of food; usually, an extra plate, sit it next to the resident and feed the resident and eat for themselves out of the other plate.

I personally dislike feeding residents.

I would rather clean poop.

It's weird, I know, but that's the thing that I dislike in nursing.

I can't explain it; there is something about feeding an adult who is spitting and drooling mashed potatoes, peas, and meat like a baby. My stomach can't take it. Think of it kind of like a person not liking clowns, hating a particular smell, afraid of squirrels; it's a quirk.

But if you ask the next nurse, she would probably rather feed a resident rather than to clean feces from a resident…we all have the quirky things that we like to do in nursing and the things that we don't want to do.

The whole assisting and feeding residents is a train wreck.

I find that this is because there are usually not enough people to help with feeding residents. If there are 110 residents, 2 nurses, and there are 10 CNAs working (good luck with seeing that number of CNAs at once), that means that each CNA is responsible for around 10-11 patients each. At mealtime, let's say ¾ of the residents are in the dining room, and the other roughly 30-40 residents remain in their rooms and have to be fed by someone.

That is a great stretch of work for the staff.

Let's then put 6 CNAs in the dining room and leave the other four on the halls. The nurses usually have to help with this chaos. I've been in nursing homes where a nursing assistant will sit and feed 2 or 3 residents at the same time with the same spoon. Management doesn't care, as long as the residents are fed.

Then after the residents are half-fed, some of the nursing assistants will eat the remaining food trays which haven't been touched, especially if it's one of the meals that they like.

Not Me....I'm picky regarding my food.

Over the years, I've had many conversations regarding myself and feeding residents. Most nurses have to "feed" when there isn't enough staff to do so.

A handful of facilities will incorporate supervised meals and feeding into the plan of care for the resident to promote a kind of bonding between the nurses and the residents.

This is just a cheap way of not hiring an adequate number of staff.

I was sitting at a table one day feeding a resident when I heard a commotion. A nursing assistant Sally was feeding residents at the table, She may have been feeding 3 people. You can imagine that the dining hall is quite large, full, and noisy at mealtimes.

From what I could make out from the commotion is that one of the residents was alert enough to tell the Sally that she didn't want to be fed with the same spoon that she had used for the other residents at the table.

The cna looked annoyed.

The resident then told her that if she put her phone away she might be able to feed everyone, individually and properly.

This was another problem in the nursing home. The constant use of cell phones by the CNAs, yes, even while feeding.

Sally continued to look annoyed.

The resident told Sally that she didn't want any of the food.

Sally jumped up, threw the residents' food tray away, and walked out of the dining hall, saying that she needed a break.

Truthfully, this was really an excuse; an excuse not to have to do any more work.

We continued to feed the residents.

One of the nurses asked the resident, whose food was thrown away if she wanted another tray of food.

She didn't answer.

She slowly wheeled herself out of the dining hall.

We all looked on.

We did nothing. We said nothing. We continued to rush through getting the other residents fed.

No point in writing her up; when attempting a write-up or any kind of disciplinary paperwork, the nursing assistant will usually offer some lame excuse for her behavior. She will get a slap on her wrist, and that's that. She might even give the nurse a smirk as she leaves the supervisor's office. As I said, no one in management "really" cares.

Sidebar, if you have ever questioned the idea of what happens with the food that you bring to the facility for your family member. The only residents that keep these things are the ones that are 100% alert, no confusion or dementia. It's usually eaten by the CNAs. The nurses will often tell the nurses' aides to put the food at the resident's bedside, and then slowly, everyone sneaks into the room to eat it. Some don't sneak; they blatantly eat the food without regard.

Sins of Nurses

"If you find it in your heart to care for somebody else, you will have succeeded."

-Maya Angelou

Chapter 27

SHOWER DAY

Today really isn't much different from any other nursing home day. It is shower day. You would be hard-pressed to find any facility in any state, which gives its residents a shower or bath every day. There is always a shower day, showers are given maybe 3 days a week in a fair facility and 4 days a week in a good facility. One of the problems is that for several reasons, the elderly have an aversion to water. I am going to assume that it has much to do with them being fragile, thin skin layers, cold water, rushed, and a nasty attitude by the CNA who is to perform this task. Many of these residents have some form of dementia and cannot verbalize accurately what they are feeling. They simply "feel" and sense certain things. Just as we can sense when we are in the store shopping, and the salesperson is having a bad day and is giving the most minimal attempt at customer service.

If a CNA is complaining, snatching, and grabbing the resident to give them a shower, they can sense this and not want to participate. On shower day, many nurses spend their time trying to convince the resident to take a shower, and the CNAs usually spend their shower day trying to get out of giving a shower. On shower day, you will find the good CNAs showering at the start of their shift. They will walk into the door giving showers. They will probably have 5-6 plus showers to provide. The good nursing assistants already know who is agreeable to taking a shower so they will get started with them right away. They will save the difficult ones for last. The bad nursing assistants will start the day off complaining about how they can't get the showers done. Then they will spend a good deal of time following the nurse around trying to get her to sign off on the paperwork, stating that the resident refused. If that doesn't work, the nursing assistant will simply grab a basin and give the resident a sponge bath. This is the most favorite option. The lousy nurse doesn't care either way, as long as they don't smell the resident, and even if they do smell the resident, it doesn't matter. I've fought many battles with nursing assistants regarding giving the residents baths. It is not unheard of for a resident to go weeks without a shower. It's one of the big problems I find in the nursing home. If nursing assistants spent more time doing work as opposed to complaining about the work, they might actually get some work done. Its 5am and its shower day. Vanessa and Sarah are doing their usual, complaining about giving showers. They are both responsible for providing 4 showers each today. I see Vanessa down the hall, she is walking towards me, and I already know how this is about to go down.

"Nurse Green, you already know that Mr. Streeter is not going to let me give him a shower today, can I just give him a bed bath? " She says to me.

"Vanessa, we've been through this every week. He needs a shower." She walks off while I'm talking to her. I see Sarah a few hours later. She comes to me to sign off on her sheet, which states that she gave showers today. I ask her directly, "Did you give all of these residents' showers today?" She looks at me with frustration....and states,

"No, I did not, I gave them all bed baths. "

Then I ask her, "If you know that today is shower day, why did you give them bed baths?" She replies, "Nurse Green, I am not about to fight with these people about giving them a shower if they don't want one. Are you going to sign off on my sheet or not? "

"No, I am not." I reply to her.

She storms off, yelling, "I am so sick and tired of you and this bullshit. You have to be difficult every single time you work; I'm going to talk to the supervisor about you."

I'm in the middle of passing out medication, but I stop and go into the room of one of her residents. "Mr. Farmington, how are you today, sir? " He states that he is okay.

"Sir, did you get a bed bath today?"

He states that he has and that he feels good today.

"Mr. Farmington, would you like to take a shower today?"

"Nooo, I already had the bed bath. " He says.

"But wouldn't you rather sit in a shower chair and sit under a nice hot shower?" I ask him.

"Well, yes, that would have been nice," He says.

I then tell him that tomorrow he will get a shower. I'm walking out of his room, taking notes.

I pass one of the resident rooms where the door is closed, and I hear Sarah on the other side of it.

"Mrs. Woods, you have to take a shower today because I don't want the fucking nurse complaining that I didn't give you a shower!"

I then hear the resident Mrs. Woods complaining.

"But I don't want a shower, it's always too cold in there, leave me alone."

I hear Sarah say to her, "I'm not playing with you today, I need my job! Get your ass up and come on to this shower room!"

I knock and enter at the same time, I want to see what she is doing, and it was just as I figured. She had the resident by the arms and was wrestling to get her into the wheelchair. She threw her into the wheelchair just as I entered the room. She looked at me and exclaimed, "See what I mean nurse, these people don't want to take showers." I then say to her that it is all in the approach. I let her know that I was outside of the door listening and that I heard Mrs. Woods complaining about it being cold. I then ask Sarah to go and to get the shower room ready and that I would bring Mrs. Woods to her, she leaves out of the room using profanity and complaining. I give Mrs. Woods a few minutes to calm down by just talking to her softly. Now that she is calm, I say to her.

"Mrs. Woods, Sarah has gone to the shower room to make sure that the heaters are on so that it won't be cold when you go in." I proceed to wheel her out of the room.

She is complaining a little bit. I go and grab a lot of towels. I'm pushing her down the hall very slow and talking to her calmly about how warm the shower room will be when we get there. We arrive at the shower room. I tell Mrs. Woods to wait for a second while I check things out. I knock, and I hear Sarah's voice. I enter. The shower is not warm; the heaters haven't been turned on. I then ask Sarah,

"If you know that she complains about being cold, why wouldn't you have the shower room warm for her?"

She exclaims, "Nurse Green, you are really irritating me today, bring her in here so that I can get this shower over with!"

I look at her with disgust. It's not new to me; this is the norm, disrespect, and laziness. I turn the shower room heaters on and walk away. I tell Mrs. Woods that the shower room is not quite ready yet. My work continues to get further behind. When I think that the room is warm, we enter. As soon as she sees Sarah, she starts to complain that she doesn't want the shower. I assure her that Sarah is going to be gentle and kind to her while giving the shower. Sarah just stares at me and rolls her eyes. I push the wheelchair toward her and say,

"If you talked to her nicely and warmed up the shower room, she would probably take a shower without a complaint."

She looks at me, "Whatever, Nurse Green, do your job, and let me do my job."

I walk out of the shower room to see one of the supervisors walking with Vanessa. This is one of the lazy supervisors who doesn't care much about much. If things look in order, that is all that matters to her. They don't actually have to be in order. I knew that Vanessa would go to her. The supervisor, Nurse Blouin, asks me if she can see me in her office for a few minutes. I tell her that I am busy, can I speak to her after I finish the medications. She says that it can't wait.

It actually can wait, but if she doesn't talk to me now, there won't be a "show" of authority for the CNAs to see. I walk down the hall to her office. Once behind closed doors, she begins by telling me that she knows that I am a hardworking and efficient nurse who likes to do things the way that they are supposed to be done, but I'm going to have to give the CNAs a break. I ask her what she means by this. She says that if I know that the CNAs have 5-6 showers to provide and they can't get to them all, just sign off on their shower sheets and say that they are done anyway.

FYI, these sheets are an indicator of care that can be looked at by other management. This is not the first time that I have been in her office. My story doesn't change much. If the CNAs made an honest attempt at care, then I would have no problem noting that. But this is not the case. I just spoke to Mr. Streeter, who got a bed bath. He would have taken a shower, he agrees to take one tomorrow, I said. I then proceed to tell her what has just happened with Mrs. Woods. *My mind is racing, I'm so sick of this bullshit.* I continue and tell her, "The CNAs simply do not want to give showers because of the work involved, we both know that. I just don't understand what you want me to do. You want the residents to have showers only on paper? Why doesn't the facility do away with having the nurse's sign for the showers and just keep a record of when the CNAs "say" that they gave the showers?" I exclaim.

"Well, the point of your signature is to show that the CNA actually gave a shower and you verified that and actually, you are the only nurse who won't sign the "shower sheets," all of the other nurses don't have a problem signing them." She explained. I just look at her and state, "I'm not signing the sheet if they aren't doing the showers!"

She then says that Vanessa and Sarah no longer want to work under my supervision and that she is going to have to switch some things around. I tell her that it will be fine. I suggest a couple of the hard-working CNAs who I know will do their work, and they don't have a problem with me. She didn't mention that she would reprimand or write up a report regarding Sarah. I wasn't surprised. She eventually switched the assignments and placed two different CNAs under my supervision. Cheryl and Sherry. They were good and didn't complain much regarding doing their work. They already knew the expectation of working with me. They weren't turning cartwheels to work with me, but they did their job, and I did mine, we all survived. I would see Vanessa and Sarah working on the other halls. Maybe I didn't look hard enough, but I don't recall ever seeing Vanessa and Sarah going anywhere near the shower room once they started working under the other nurse. I heard many negative things that were said about me, from the CNAs and the other nurses. Everything from, "She wants to be a supervisor" to "Someone should give her a button that says super nurse" or "Ms. Perfect nurse."

…. I hope that you get the points in this story on how the system fails and why nurses tolerate what we tolerate. It's usually a losing battle. I've found that it is easier to get rid of a nurse who "bucks" the system than to get rid of a bad CNA. After all, a bad CNA is better than no CNA. Nursing assistants are usually hard to come by and to keep. If they have to let someone go, that someone is going to be the LPN.

Sins of Nurses

"You cannot open a book without learning something."

-Confucius

Chapter 28

EXPLOITATION

Hardly anybody talks about the exploitation of nurses brought to the U.S. from other countries. I have heard from other nurses and have seen for myself how this exploitation sometimes works. One such story went as follows, I was working at a nursing home, and I couldn't help but notice that this dilapidated "Hell hole" had an unusually high number of Asian nurses. They seemed to have a minimal grasp of the English language, seemingly new to the United States. I remember one of the nurses kept trying to ask me about a medicine. She was grossly mispronouncing its name, and we were having a difficult time trying to understand each other. We eventually managed to figure things out.

These Asian nurses were working throughout this building. As I went throughout my day at one point, I heard one of the nurses say that she was going upstairs to get something to eat. I thought that I must have misunderstood her because, although this was a newly converted 6-story building, there were only patients on the first three floors. There was storage and renovations on the other three floors. (so I thought)no food vending or soda machines.

She couldn't be going upstairs to any place, as there was no upstairs to go to. Then one of the nurses told me that the Asian nurses were living on the top floors of this nursing home.

"What do you mean they live on the top floors?" I asked.

She asked me not to repeat anything as she spoke to me in a very low tone, almost whispering.

She began by telling me that the top two floors housed a dormitory-style of living and that nurses were living there. Many from Asia, mostly from the Philippines. She told me that many had contracts, which kept them employed with this nursing home for up to 5 years.

Their pay was nominal compared to the U.S registered and licensed practical nurses. They lived the first 6-9 months or so in the building; after this, they could look for apartments or other housing as long as it was close to the facility, and they could be reached at all times.

Only in the U.S !!

Throughout my nursing career i had heard similar stories before.

I have to admit that the housing part of this story was a bit different from what I had heard about these nurses previously. These foreign nurses and others that I had met were usually unhappy with these contractual arrangements. Often, they were registered nurses in their country, that were marketed to and promised things by American recruiters from private facilities.

These particular nurses' came from Asia with big dreams. These dreams didn't meet the hype.

I really felt sorry for these nurses for a while, until they started to change. They slowly became what I call "Americanized," meaning that they soon adapted and adopted the American way of nursing.

Compared to the way that they treated each other and their thoughts regarding family, it was odd to see that they had little respect and compassion for our elderly, American elders.

They talked to each other, they spent much time together, they looked out for each other, they ate together and even slept together.

The other thing is, they had little regard or respect for American nurses as if we were to blame for their circumstances in some way.

They simply did their jobs and were minimally polite to us. Mostly speaking to each other in their native languages as though we weren't around.

It was damned annoying.

Would it surprise you to know that they don't care for American patients to the best of their abilities?

But then they are following our examples; they have a great point of reference. The way in which we take care of our own.

It was an evening shift, and I had received report from the nurse I was relieving. She was Filipino and had struggled a bit, but we managed to get through the change of shift report.

I was pushing my cart down the hall and I heard two people yelling loudly in English and another language. I walked into a room and there was a Filipino nurse and a Filipino nursing assistant standing over one of the residents. The resident was trying to move her chair but she couldn't. The CNA was standing behind the chair holding it and the nurse was standing in front of the chair straddling the patient's legs, which kept her from moving. The patient was cursing, swinging her arms and legs and yelling that she wasn't taking any medicine from the nurse. She seemed to think that the nurse was trying to kill her. This wasn't unusual. Many dementia patients had similar thoughts at times. A notion that nurses and cna's were trying to harm them. This had nothing to do with race or origin. The CNA was saying something to the nurse in her language.

"Hey, you need some help? " I asked.

"I need some help; they won't let me leave, call the police!" the patient yelled.

The nurse began to yell at the resident.

"You have to take your medicine! Just take your medicine," the nurse yells.

She then begins to speak to the CNA in their native language.

"You have to take your medicine, take it!" She yells at the patient again, laughing.

She then grabs her nose and attempts to force the crushed medicine in her mouth with the spoon. The patient spits out the medicine and hits the nurse.

This Filipino nurse hits her back.

The patient hits the nurse again.

They both laugh.

They look over at me, then turn away and begin to speak so that I don't understand them. They both laugh again. The CNA jokingly hits the resident on her arm. The patient hits her.

They begin to speak in their language again, laughing loudly.

I look on.

"you know that ...."

I was going to say something, I changed my mind. I walked out of the room. I continued passing out my medication. I didn't have time to fight with another nurse; I had my own problems and work to do. I pushed my cart down the hall.

Sins of Nurses

"In a world filled with hate, we must still dare to hope. In a world filled with anger, we must still dare to comfort. In a world filled with despair, we must still dare to dream. And in a world filled with distrust, we must still dare to believe."

– Michael Jackson

Chapter 29

SMH

I was sitting in the staff dining room when the Director of Nursing announced overhead that all nurses should report to their stations for a special meeting with her.

I thought to myself, *what is going on now*? The Director was informing everyone that JCAHO or Joint Commission on Accreditation of Healthcare Organizations would be in the building tomorrow.

"Oh shit," I thought to myself, actually, I had said it aloud, and everyone had laughed.

We all knew that this was very serious and that there was nothing to laugh about. It was just my luck that I was scheduled to be working at this nursing home for the rest of this week. This SHIT HOLE! I was going to have to be stuck here during the inspection by JCAHO. The only thing I would have in my favor is my ability to say that I was not regular staff and had only worked a few times in this facility. I wasn't familiar with "all" of their policies and procedures should I be hung up on something that they might ask me. I would still have to know basic facility competencies to get through this inspection. I wondered how this facility would be able to pass any type of inspection. There were two floors, and each floor had about 70 patients with 2 nurses and about 6 CNAs who had 10-12 patients each. The facility was dirty, most of the residents didn't have adequate linens for their beds, and the CNAs complained that they never had towels and supplies to take care of the residents. The place was a train wreck. Again, how were they going to pass? But honestly, I'd seen just as bad, if not worst, other nursing homes pass these inspections, usually through some form of trickery. The hustling and bustling had begun to get things in order before the inspectors arrive the next morning. It was going to be a long day tomorrow, noooo......a long day today. I managed to get through my day. It was hell. All in preparation to make sure we had maintained a certain standard of care in this nursing home. What a joke! I finally went home and tried to sleep that night. I could lose my license working at that place. I was tempted to call off. I needed the money; I was divorced with three children and could not miss any pay dates on my paycheck. I arrived slightly earlier than my shift was to start on the next day. I wanted to familiarize myself with the cart a bit more and my surroundings. The first thing I notice when I enter my unit is that it smells clean. Someone must have cleaned all night in order for it to smell like this. The next thing I notice is that there are three medication carts instead of two. I put my things into a locker and when I return there are two nurses sitting at the nurses' station and the unit manager begins to explain to me that there will be three of us working and that the assignment sheets and carts have all been prepared to accommodate this. I'm shaking my head. I walk down the halls to the resident rooms and notice that there are new looking, fresh linens on all of the beds. I continue to shake my head. I see one of the certified nursing assistants, and I ask her what is going on. She starts laughing and begins to tell me that she has been working at this nursing home for almost 10 years and that this is what happens when management knows that JCAHO is coming into the building. I ask her, "But where did all of this linen come from? I know they didn't buy all of this last night!" She laughs more and states, "Of course not." She walks me into a room and closes the door. She then grabs a piece of wood that is under the bed, pulls out a chair, and pokes the wood to the ceiling, lifting up one of the squares. There is a big plastic bag there. She pulls it down and opens it for me; the bag contains a practically new blanket, sheets, towels and a few other toiletries. All hidden in this bag, hidden in this ceiling. I know this sounds made up but it's not. I shake my head. "You have to be kidding me?" I walk back down the hall to the nurses' station. The nursing assistants are waiting at the desk for their assignments. I want to faint. They never do this! They know when jobs and paychecks are on the line, I suppose. No rude, ignorant behavior today. I wasn't surprised. Instead of there being the usual 7-8, nursing assistants, there were 10.

WOW!!

I couldn't help but laugh again. Each nursing assistant will now have a more reasonable 6-7 resident each that they are responsible for. The nursing assignment is divided so that two of us will have 20 residents each, and the third nurse who is regular staff will have about 30 residents. I start down the hall to begin my morning med pass. I look down the hall and notice that there are 3 people in business casual with clipboards and pens. They are here. They walk through the rooms, talk to some of the residents, talk to staff, management is not far behind. Management is watching for any signs that there is a problem. The surveyors are looking for things like adequate staffing to care for the number of residents on the floor, adequate nursing coverage, they have even been known to do something like slide a piece of paper with a time on it…under a resident sheet. They will return to check the resident in two hours. This is what is considered the standard. Every resident is checked every two hours, and if they are bed-bound, they should be turned. If they are not turned, they will not pass the test of the inspector. All of the nursing assistants are aware of this trick. On this day, every resident will be checked, turned, fed, showered, medicated, and anything else that they could need while the surveyors are in the building. Knowing when JCAHO is coming makes all the difference in whether a facility will pass this accreditation. All facilities are aware of the window in which the surveyors will come. They can usually narrow it down to within a month. If you know someone or pay someone, you will know within 24 hrs. If you've ever wondered why there is no real change in the state of nursing home care, this is a significant factor. Real change may come if the nursing home doesn't know when they are to be inspected. Enough failures across the states will help a great deal in the monitoring of these rat holes that should be closed down.

I'm back at the nurses' station, and I am doing some charting. One of the surveyors walks up to me and starts asking me questions. She asks me if there is any information regarding this facility that I would like to disclose to her. I think hard for a minute, and then I look at her.

"No, ma'am."

Sins of Nurses

"Real knowledge is to know the extent of one's ignorance."

-Confucius

Chapter 30

NARCOTICS AND MEDICATIONS ARE FOR THE PATIENTS?

There have been many stories of narcotic and medication abuse by nurses; I don't think I've ever known of such a story that wasn't true. I'm not saying that there has never been a false accusation, but just that usually when nurses see SIGNS of drug abuse in another nurse, there is probably something to it. Nurses who abuse narcotics commonly abuse other things, not just legal drugs. I have encountered many nurses in my career that I thought was using some kind of drug. This is something that is hard to prove. No employer is going to accuse or even drug test a nurse without adequate suspicion. Even then, it might not happen. Even a Nurse stealing medicine is not a new occurrence.

I remember one such incident where two nurses were covering for each other and stealing medication. They started somewhat subtle at first, and then they became very bold, so bold that figuring out which medicines they were stealing had become very apparent. One day you were working your shift, and you knew that there was a huge bottle of Tylenol with 1000 pills on the cart, and the next day the bottle would be almost empty. One day you would check cards of stock medications, and then the next day, many cards would be gone. We started noticing a pattern of large amounts of medicine disappearing when these two particular nurses would work on the weekend. It's Saturday, it's laid back, not too many people around. I suppose someone could easily take medicine out of the building then. I remember working on a Friday, checking medicines, and then writing down the number of cards for each. (Just to prove to others and myself that we weren't imagining disappearing medication.) I recall that a large amount of medication was no longer on the cart when I returned on Monday. Just to see if I were correct in my suspicions, I went to the medication "closet" to check those medications, as well. I was amazed at the amount of medicine that was missing. A stock medication card may hold as few as 30 pills or up to 90 pills. I recall that there seemed to be pain pills such as Tylenol, Motrin, and Tramadol missing. Antibiotics such as Penicillin, Doxycycline, Amoxicillin, were also missing. Even some blood pressure pills such as Lisinopril and Hydrochlorothiazide were missing.

I wasn't the only nurse who suspected these two particular nurses that were stealing. Most of us joked that we believed that these two nurses must have had a side hustle {or something like one} and that they were selling medications out of the trunk of their cars. We also noticed that these two nurses seemed to give an awful lot of narcotics when they worked; Far more than the rest of us. Many nurses know that it is easy to steal narcotics if you really want to. For instance, one such way would be to pretend to give doses when you really do not. A patient might have scheduled doses of a narcotic every 6 hours, but when you go in to give it, they will let you know that they feel fine and don't need it. A nurse who steals medication could then keep this medicine for herself. Another way might be to give a person two Tylenol instead of two similar-looking narcotic pills, such as Percocet. Most patients usually won't know the difference because the pills look pretty similar. If you are determined to steal narcotics and/or any medication, it is easy. I cannot say how often this occurs, but I can say that it definitely does occur.

I once read a newspaper article that involved a nurse who would steal the pain patches of morphine from patients and use them on herself. I remember working one day, and my supervisor had decided that he was going to finally {after many complaints} try to put a stop to the nurses who were stealing the medication. He waited close to the end of the shift to approach us, nurses, on the large number of medications that seemed to be missing each week. It was Beatrice and myself working. We were about an hour away from the end of our shift and were making sure that our carts and charting were in order. Juan, our supervisor, approached us while we were in the medication room and asked us both to step back from the carts. He then proceeded to give us a lecture on how stealing would no longer be tolerated and that if nurses were stealing, they would be terminated.

What are you telling us for? The thieves aren't here today, I thought to myself. After he spoke for a while, he then said to us that if we had currently, on this day, taken any medications, we should admit this now.

I started laughing. I thought it was funny. I shook my head and said, "Sorry, I'm not hiding any medicine, and I have nothing to hide." I then threw my hands up.

Beatrice began to cry and apologize.

I thought she was joking! She then walked over to the medication cart and went to the bottom of the cart. There she pulled out its bottom-most drawer, got down on her knees, and pulled out several cards of medication that she had hidden underneath the drawer. She handed these cards to Juan. Juan and I both looked shocked. I think Juan looked shocked that she had admitted to anything. I looked shocked *because who does that*? I knew that no one would have ever thought to look under the bottom drawer for medications. Not to mention that she wasn't even the type of nurse who stole anything. *So I thought.* I guess she could have been on that TV show about dumb criminals. I would have thought that she would have simply put the medications back where she had gotten them and simply stopped stealing. *Go figure.* No one would have been the wiser. I don't think that anyone ever even thought of her as that type of Nurse. But here she was admitting that she had stolen medicines, where she had put them and was handing them over.

WOW!

Juan then walked her to his office. He closed the door; I don't recall seeing her come out of his office. I did see her as she left the building. We were parked next to each other.

"It was nice working with you," she said, without looking up.

"Same here."

I later heard that she had been suspended. However, she never did return. What was odd is that this wasn't one of the two nurses that we all knew to be stealing medications! The other two continued to steal for a while. They did seem to slow down on the amount of medication that they were stealing. Eventually, they both resigned and left before they were caught in the act.

Sins of Nurses

"Nothing in the world is more dangerous than sincere ignorance and conscientious stupidity."

ML King, Jr.

Chapter 31

EVERYONE KNOWS ABOUT LORIN

Lorin is about 5'10, 32 years old; she has curly light red hair, she is medium build, and married with three children. I really like her. She has a great sense of humor and knows how to make you laugh. She seems to know her shit when it comes to nursing.

I don't think that I would trust her with MY life, but she's okay.

There is just one thing about her ....and everybody knows about it.

Lorin steals narcotics.

I guess we don't know factually, but we are pretty damned sure.

She always seems to be tired and nodding off.

She seems to always be generally "off."

Don't ask me to try and explain "off." It's that sense that something is not quite right with her. One thing for sure is that whenever she works, the narcotic count seems to always be "off" by one or two pills. All of us nurses had begun to watch her.

As a matter of fact, last week, two nurses got into a big argument because the narcotic count was off again. Joan had relieved Lorin the night before, but today Marcy was relieving Joan, and she noticed a discrepancy in the narcotic count.

What are you talking about?" says Marcy

"Are you saying that I use drugs?" says Joan

"I'm not accusing you of using drugs; I'm saying that since the alprazolam is missing, we have to call the manager! Can you account for it or not? "*says Marcy*

"What would I do with the pill?!" *says Joan*

"I don't know, and I don't care, I'm just saying that the count is off! Either you gave the pill, or you just don't know where it is…if you didn't give it, and you don't know where it is, I'm calling the unit manager!" *says Marcy*

"And what are you going to tell her?" *says Joan*

"Joan, get out of my face, I'm done with this conversation." *Yells Marcy.*

Marcy gets up and grabs the phone to call the manager. Joan walks away, pissed.

Lorin happens to be sitting at the nurses' station, shuffling papers, and listening to the whole thing. A couple of the nursing assistants are sitting there as well.

Amazing! All the work that needs to be done and CNA's seem to find the time to sit more than the nurses.

Sometimes I think the nursing station should be called the "nursing assistants station."

Anyway, back to Lorin.

Lorin's' shift has ended, and she should have been gone 30 minutes ago. She is still here, sitting and listening.

I stood at my med cart, watching the whole thing shaking my head. I couldn't believe that they were arguing like that. I glance over at Lorin; she looks over at me she then shook her head at me, shrugged her shoulders and smiled As if to say, "those poor nurses arguing like that."

I laughed to myself.

They both knew that Lorin had been on that cart the night before.

Joan is lazy and had probably half counted narcotics with Lorin the night prior, her BAD.

Marcy, on the other hand, is very thorough, and nothing gets past her. Your shit had better be together if she is relieving you. Joan slipped up, and Marcy caught the mistake.

Ironically, I don't get the argument.

I've had conversations with both Marcy and Joan on separate occasions, and it's very clear.

EVERYONE KNOWS ABOUT LORIN! EVERYONE!!

So while they were arguing with each other, it was misdirected.

Joan and Marcy were called to the office of the Director of Nursing. I'm not sure what happened. They barely talked to each other after that.

Lorin didn't seem to steal a particular type of narcotic. It was anything controlled.

It could be anything from Oxycodone, Dilaudid, Norco, Alprazolam, Tramadol, Ambien, Percocet, Vicodin, even fentanyl patches would come up wasted.

It didn't seem to matter, as long as it was a narcotic.

So how was she doing it?

Well, we noticed that it seemed as though she started off very subtly by doing things like "dropping" a narcotic and having to waste it (throw it away) to get another one. No one actually saw her ever throw away a pill; she always said things like, "I'll throw it away in a second."

Someone would then co-sign with her, that they saw her drop and then discard the pill.

We were all noticing that she was always asking you to co-sign a "wasted" medication with her. She was always asking you to do this after the fact. You didn't see her drop and/or waste anything. She would just tell you something like "Hey, I dropped a pill, can you sign the waste with me?" most of us would simply just sign.

Then we noticed that it seemed that after she worked, many of the residents appeared to be in more pain than usual. Trust me, we had enough residents in the nursing home who were addicted to their narcotics.

Her not giving them didn't go unnoticed by us and definitely not by particular residents.

"You know, I'm really hurting; It seems like my pills didn't kick in at all last night." says a resident who loves her Dilaudid.

We simply started to notice the pattern of the residents complaining about being in pain after she worked.

Eventually, she stepped things up a notch.

You know how the narcotic drawer can be filled with narcotics from residents who've left and gone home, or they were discontinued for one reason or another?

And you still have to keep counting all of it?

Well, she began to destroy the narcotics that were on her cart and, at times, the cart of her coworkers.

So you're working, and here she comes. "Hey, do you have any narcotics that you want to destroy?"

"Yeah, a drawer full."

"Okay, I can destroy them for you." (this is at a time when most facilities didn't require two nurses to witness the destruction of narcotics. As long as the nurse was a Registered nurse, that was the only requirement.)

We then account for all of the narcotics together, sign everything that would be destroyed - because you need two signatures. Then when it came time to destroy them, she would quickly walk away toward the med room to destroy them without you.

"I got it; I'll just be in here destroying these."

At this time, facilities would destroy narcotics by punching out each pill and placing them into the sharps container. Sometimes we would crush them and then flush the powder down the toilet or pour them down the sink. Getting them taken off the cart and not having to count them every shift was the only thing we cared about in the beginning.

So into the med room, she would go with cards of narcotics to destroy.

No one really thought too much about it initially, but then we all started to think about it.

I think someone eventually brought this to the attention of management.

They knew what was happening, as it was the buzz of the facility, but management was reluctant to make the accusation directly.

Eventually, our facility implemented a policy that only managers could destroy narcotics. They were to be collected and given to that units manager, who would then destroy the medications at some point. Nowadays, facilities send them back to the pharmacy for a credit.

This stopped that little routine of Lorin getting large numbers of narcotics.

Lorin was then back to her old way of stealing narcotics. Every nurse knew to thoroughly count her medications when Lorin was involved.

Even if the narcotic count was correct, you went behind Lorin to double-check things. She seemed to have stopped for a while, but we knew she was doing something.

After she would leave the building, usually, we would look at the narcotic book to protect ourselves and to make sure you hadn't missed anything. There was always something interesting to find.

Residents who never took narcotics at all would have taken their oxycodone or morphine or whatever pill during the night when she worked.

We would find it and then laugh. "There it is!"

We knew that this was "really" no joking matter, but we couldn't help it. The Unit Manager and the Director of Nursing knew what was going on. Holly, one of the other nurses, had said that {management said} that they couldn't single her out for drug testing without any real proof. I guess the speculation of 4 or 5 nurses wasn't enough.

They didn't want to know.

They liked Lorin, so they chose to ignore all the gossip and speculations. Lorin's behavior continued for months.

Then one day, Lorin's stealing narcotics' was to end. One of the nurses was looking in the narcotic book after Lorin left and noticed that Lorin had "wasted" 3 pills during the night. Next to the sign out for one pill, Lorin had initialed, and so had the other nurse. That was about 1am.

Then around 4am, the same thing happened. Two pills "wasted" this time.

The problem for Lorin is that, although she worked that night with Nancy and Nancy had co-signed the wasted pills, Nancy was the nurse reading the book, and she had not signed nor "wasted" anything with Lorin. She turned three shades of red. "That is not my signature, I didn't sign that, I didn't waste anything with her!" We all stared at each other. Nancy took the book and marched into the Director of Nurses' office. They fired Lorin for forgery.

Sins of Nurses

"I've learned that people will forget what you said, people will forget what you did, but people will never forget how you made them feel." -Maya Angelou

Chapter 32

THAT WAS MEAN

I'm working at this nursing home. I don't think I had been there more than 2 or 3 times. I was there through a nursing agency. It was an evening shift, and I was down the hall, passing medication when I hear yelling. It was probably around 8pm.

I knew the nursing assistants were getting the residents ready for bed. I figured it was probably coming from one of the ones who didn't want to get undressed or simply didn't want to go to bed.

"Stop saying that, you're telling a lie!"

"He would never do that!"

I looked down the hall and saw a female resident standing with three nursing assistants around her. I walked down to get a better grasp of what was going on.

Knowing the nursing assistants, something was happening that shouldn't be.

This came to be my perception of most nursing assistants, always doing something that they shouldn't be.

There they all were, sitting and laughing.

There was Mrs. Herring with her coat and purse, refusing to go to bed and saying that she was going home to her husband.

They were telling her that her husband didn't want her anymore. That he had a new girlfriend and that there was no point in her trying to go home.

They were all laughing.

She may have been confused, but somehow she knew that what they were saying was not true. She may have had dementia, but she knew that the man that she had married and loved for over 50 years was not with another woman. Actually, her husband was dead.

My understanding is that she had never come to accept this and that the facility and family members had given up on trying to get her to understand. She was trying to do what she had always done, go home to her husband.

"Your husband doesn't want you no more, we already told you. He has a new girlfriend" one cna said

She became very angry at this and was yelling at them to stop saying this. They thought it to be hilarious.

I had heard enough, I intervened. "What are you all doing?"

"Just playing around with Mrs. Herring," another said.

"She doesn't seem to be laughing; cut it out, please!" I said.

One of the CNAs mumbled something, and they all started to laugh.

"Come on Mrs. Herring." I began to walk her back to her room.

"Why don't you get into bed now, I'm sure Hulbert will be here to visit with you tomorrow." She seemed to feel better. Getting her to take her coat off and go to bed wasn't exactly an easy task, so I left her sitting on her bed, coat, and purse in hand. I walked back to where the nursing assistants were seated, of course, no one had moved, they were still there laughing at the incident. I reminded them of what they already knew to be as unacceptable behavior; I told them that what they were doing was considered abuse, and if I thought it would do any good, I would write them all up. They began to argue and get loud with me.

Their behavior was so outlandish, unprofessional, and disrespectful. As I walked away, they continued.

Someone called me a bitch! I could hear them laughing. I decided to write each of them up anyway. I wrote my incident report regarding what had happened, and then I slid my report under the door of the director of nursing. I was sure I would have drama when I returned tomorrow for my 3-11pm shift, but I didn't care. I received a call about 11am advising that the facility had requested that I not return because of my behavior.

Not surprised.

I probed into what was meant by "my behavior."

I was told that the three nursing assistants whom I had written my reports on had written their own reports. They had stated in their reports that I was rude, unprofessional, and had been this way to the residents.

They had all observed my behavior and had spoken to ME about my behavior.

They told me that they were going to be reporting me and that I must have reported them falsely before they had time to submit their reports. I laughed to myself. No one asked me anything, no one wanted to hear my side of the story. The agency that I worked for told me not to worry about it. They would find another assignment for me. I wasn't shocked, this had happened on other occasions. This kind of incident is what keeps nurses from saying anything about the CNAs. The facilities really don't want to hear the truth when it comes to these things. It is easier to ask one nurse from an agency not to return, rather than to fire or reprimand 3 much-needed nursing assistants.

Sins of Nurses

"Loneliness and the feeling of being unwanted is the most terrible poverty."

-Mother Teresa

Chapter 33 .

THE BATTERED PIMP

When I met, Joe he was probably in his 60's and was known by all the nurses and CNAs as a pimp who we all felt got what he deserved. He had contractures and deformities about his head. He had two large wounds, one to his butt and another to his hip and a few small ones. He was no longer able to walk and was barely able to talk. What he could say was barely discernable. You could make out only a word here and there. Usually, "fuck you" was pretty clear.

Joe had been beaten with a bat that had left him broken and paralyzed, his body riddled with wounds that wouldn't heal and some brain damage. He was in a room by himself because he was on contact isolation for MRSA.

These wounds required daily dressing changes. Anyone entering the room would need to wear a gown, gloves, and a mask to protect him or herself. No one wanted to go in and take care of him because many times, he would spit on you, pinch you, throw feces on you, or worse grab you.

If he got those claws into you, it would be hell getting away, and you could have a potential scratch filled with feces and infection. Frequently most of us were hit or spit on by Joe.

One night I was working the night shift with two of the male CNAs Marcus and Jason. I was sitting at the nurses' station waiting for the CNAs to get Joe ready for me so that I could do his treatments. This meant undressing him, turning him on his side, and holding him down so that I could do his wound care.

I'm outside of his door, putting on what feels like riot gear just to go in and do these dressing changes. I was irritated with dealing with him tonight, he had been in rare form. Yelling, spitting, you name it.

He could be quite alert at times, his mind wasn't totally gone. A few days ago, while I was doing his dressing change, the guys were joking with him and asking him questions, and one of the questions was if Joe thought I was attractive. He replied yes, the next question was, "what would you do to her if you were able to?" and his response was "fuck her to death"......no way did he just say that. But he had. The male nursing assistants thought that it was quite funny. I didn't find it funny, I guess because a small part of me was afraid of him. Whenever you went into the room the way, he stared at you. Sometimes it seemed creepy and a bit evil looking. Then other times, it appeared to be very sexual, and he would have an erection while you were there trying to give him medication. Most of the female nurses hated going into his room.

What was he thinking, this old battered pimp?

Anyway, fast forward to today and having to change his dressing. I'm putting on my riot gear to enter the room.

The two cna's are waiting for me, standing back laughing and talking shit to Joe.

I walk over to Joe and just as the guys go to turn him on his side, (it happened so quickly).

He ripped off the dressing from his hip that is saturated with foul-smelling green and yellow drainage, urine, and poop and throws it. It lands on the side of my face.

"Oh, shit" did this infected gauze just slap me in the face?

I stumbled back almost falling, Jason caught me. I let out a scream. I wasn't hurt. I was disgusted!

I immediately ran to the bathroom so that I could wash my face.

Before I could get out of the room, I could hear Marcus and Jason yelling at him. "You crippled motherfucker! You are going to pay for doing that to the nurse."

I could hear thumping sounds. I knew they were probably hitting him. The water was running, I kept running looking in the mirror at my face. I didn't look toward Joe. I did nothing, and at that moment I didn't care.

Sins of Nurses

"Nearly all men can stand adversity, but if you want to test a man's character, give him power."

-Abraham Lincoln

Chapter 34

WHEN THEY WANT YOU GONE

As always, I had high hopes for this Nursing home; they gave a great presentation as to what you could expect working there. They had a no-nonsense approach to things; they knew that there were problems with nursing assistants as there were everywhere, and they were combating this problem head-on as best they could.

Yesss, finally, a place to work in peace! So I thought.

They had a strict no cell phone policy, which was great because it was probably the #2 problem in most nursing homes.

I didn't have to work too many shifts to realize that this beautiful facility was no different from the rest. But then that's not a new concept.

Nice presentations, bad management and staff.....

The staffing person had placed me on the 2nd floor to work most of my shifts. It didn't take me more than a minute to realize that the 2nd floor had two problems.

Cam and Zolita, the two regular cna's who worked on that floor.

Zolita was relatively quiet around me; I think she was trying to figure me out.

Cam, on the other hand, didn't care. She was going to be who she was and continue to do whatever she wanted. After all, the facility let her wear several different hats. This allowed her to "get in" with upper management, which would enable them to see her exactly as SHE wanted them to see her.

Not the sneaky, unprofessional, lazy, manipulator that she was.

First problem: Run in with Zolita regarding her cell phone; problems with her the whole day being on her phone despite my asking her politely to be a bit more discreet with its use WHEN YOU KNOW YOU SHOULDN'T BE ON IT AT ALL !! eventually, I had to write her up.

This didn't sit well with Cam.

How dare I come to work at this facility and write someone up, especially her friend. *Is what I'm sure she was thinking.*

After that, Zolita stayed away from me, never a word, never a snide remark. We were nonexistent to each other.

Cam was different, she had a problem with me, and it was going to be a problem for me when she finished.

Cam stepped onto the elevator with me one day*; it was just she and I ……* she began to talk to herself, out loud

"I don't play with people!" *Indirectly meant for me,*

"people better not play with me……." I tuned her out.

I spoke to the unit manager regarding my having to write up Zolita over the weekend and that I felt that I might have problems with the two of them. *(I didn't know that she was a personal friend of Cam and Zolita's, she was their friend more than she was the unit manager*).

She assured me that she would support me regarding being their supervisor; she also informed me that I should watch them carefully as they tend to leave the unit quite frequently together and also take their lunches together, leaving their "halls" uncovered.

I'm working and they are doing just as she said, leaving the unit together and expecting that the cna from the other hall will cover their patients and their own.

Normally, two cna's that work on the same hall wouldn't leave the floor at the same time, but these two did.

The first time I noticed them leaving, I ignored them as I was very busy.

The second time.

"excuse me, are you both leaving the unit together?" I asked.

"yes, like we always do!" replied Cam smartly.

"the unit manager says that you guys shouldn't be leaving the floor together, and that one of you should stay back to answer patient call lights." I say

Cam starts to get loud and states that she is going to "ask" the Unit manager about this matter because their leaving the unit together had never been a problem before.

Cam sees the Unit manager and heads straight toward her.

I ignore her and keep working.

I then think about it and decide to listen to the question, conversation vs accusation. I head toward them and arrive just in time to hear LaVonne, the Unit Manager, telling them to go ahead to lunch, as usual. I look at her in disbelief as Cam and Zolita march past me.

Cam said something smart regarding me being a troublemaker.

I ignore her and continue straight toward Lavonne, I look at her with a question mark attached to my face.

I don't have to say a word, LaVonne looks at me and flatly reinterates that it was acceptable that they go to lunch together as long as "someone" was covering their hall.

She quickly looks away. I could see the guilt in her face.

It's a common problem. Do managers choose to face off with Nurses or CNA'S.

I can tell you, they would rather face off with nurses all day long.

But Is she serious? I'm in disbelief.

I walk away in anger, focusing on calming down instead of this foolishness.

Eventually, I see LaVonne alone in the nurses' station. I decide to confront her on her backstabbing me earlier.

"Hey, LaVonne, am I losing it, or did I miss something in our earlier conversation this morning? Because you clearly told me to watch Cam and Zolita and to monitor them leaving the unit ! I did just that, but when they got upset and confronted you, you denied having said this.

Is there some reason you changed things up and chose to not have my back?"

For a few minutes, she stammered and stuttered about what she said and implied that I misunderstood her.

I hadn't misunderstood her. Not one bit!

What LaVonne had now done was create an unnecessary problem for me. She had made it become personal-in the eyes of Zolita and Cam.

I was pissed. The disrespect and insubordination was about to increase.

This was now to be Nurse Green against the CNA'S.

If you know anything about nursing assistants, then you know that this was going to be bad for me.

I attempt to complete my shift without an incident.

I tell Cam that I need her assistance to hold a resident while I perform wound care on her butt.

"no rush, but when you go in to do your next check and change on her let me know." She ignores me and keeps walking.

It is getting closer to the end of the shift and I've been behind throughout the day.

I suddenly remember that Cam hasn't come to me regarding the resident that I have to do the wound care on.

"Hey Cam, have you changed Mrs. Polen? I need to do her dressing?"

"I've already done her!" she snaps

"But you didn't tell me that you were going to go and change her."

"well I've already changed her, and I don't have time to go back in there, I don't know what to tell you." She walks away.

I haven't done any of my treatments. I've been so busy. No point in going back to LaVonne. She would be useless.

I go to Arianna, the RN Manager, on the 2nd floor. I tell her that I have to do a treatment on Mrs. Polen and that Cam was to assist me and that she purposely avoided letting me know that she was working with Mrs. Polen and that she (Cam)is now refusing to assist me.

"well, tell her that she has to."says Arianna

" I've tried that. You're going to have to talk to her" I say.

Arianna goes to talk to Cam.

I see Arianna leaving the room where she and Cam had been speaking.

"she's ready whenever you are," Arianna says.

I grab my supplies and go into the room to do the treatment on Mrs. Polen. Cam is there waiting. I walk over to Mrs. Polen, and Cam mumbles something under her breath….

"fucking petty……."

I ignore her ugliness (inside and out.)

I complete the dressing change and hurry to the Nurses station where my relief Nurse is waiting to receive a report from me.

I exclaim to her that I am behind and that I didn't get to 3 of the treatments.

She says, "no worries. I'll take care of them for you."

"Thanks I appreciate it."

I can't wait to leave this floor. The next day I'm working on the 1st floor, and I receive a phone call from Arianna, the Manager on the second floor.

She wants to question me about some things that I neglected to do on yesterday.

"Like?" I ask her.

"well, mainly, there were some treatments that weren't done." She says.

As if I don't know where this is coming from.

Cam and Zolita knew that I hadn't finished all of my work, so they called themselves reporting me to the manager.

But as I told Arianna, "you're correct I didn't get to finish all of my work but if you look in the computer you will see my notes that I did not do them and that I endorsed them to the second shift nurse who said that she WOULD do them."

I guess you didn't look at the progress notes before you called me. BITCH!

I knew where she was going with this. But I was too smart for them. CYOB. On another day, I might have just charted that I had done these things even if I had not. But because I knew that they didn't like me, I made sure not to give them any grounds to hold anything against me. Shame on Arianna for playing into that drama and attempting to give me a "teachable moment." To satisfy her cna's.

This is that typical shit nurses have to deal with when they get on the wrong side of things with the cna's.

It is the reason why many nurses simply look the other way with cna's. They know that a cna can make you miserable and get you in a lot of trouble.

That is, if you aren't smart.

I take that back, even if you are smart, if the cna's are determined to get rid of you, you might as well quit.

I find that with nursing assistants you have to give them a taste of their own medicine, most times, in order to keep them from scaring you off!

and if they don't mind the drama, nor do I mind dishing it.

I visit the staffing coordinator later that day and tell her that I won't work on the second floor anymore.

Between the two unit managers and the nursing assistants, I just don't have time for the unnecessary drama.

I return to my work on the 1st floor for an uneventful shift.

Eventually, and within a few days and thanks to Cam.

The nursing assistants on the 1st floor have decided that they don't like me.

The usual drama ensues, cell phone use, leaving the unit, nursing assistants in the nurses station more than the nurse, profanity, loud, and unprofessional behavior.

The normal day to day activity for skilled nursing facilities cna's.

I give up attempting to gain control of the floor by speaking to the other nurse that I'm working with. If the two nurses working together were on the same page and attempting to control the floor. There might be some organization. But if your partner nurse appears used to it and doesn't seem to mind you don't stand a chance.

The cna's are pretty much staying away from me, they've heard about me and I guess its just as well.

I'm "over" all of them and their disgusting behaviors.

I'm working a double shift this day, leaving the 1st floor and headed to the 3rd floor. I leave my nursing bag at the nurses station and run to the third floor to let the nurse there know that I will be there as soon as I give report on the 1st floor.

She is ok with that so I head back down stairs to give report to the nurse on the 1st floor.

I give her report, grab my nursing bag, my clipboard and head upstairs to work my second shift on the third floor.

Around 7pm I head outside to sit in my car for my supper break.

I'm next to my car but I can't seem to find my car keys. I search everywhere. My pockets, my bag, around the car, back at the nursing cart, the bathroom on both floors, the nursing stations. My fellow nurse coworkers are looking. Security is looking, no keys anywhere.

I KNOW THAT I PUT THEM IN MY BAG!

Let's take a wild guess. CNA'S !!!

My guess is that one of those petty, unprofessional, ugly, lazy nursing assistants figured that they would teach me a lesson by taking my keys *AND THEY DID*!

I called my insurance company, they sent out a tow truck. The driver got me in my car, I knew the keys wouldn't be inside but I looked anyway.

They weren't there.

The security guy searched the grounds, no keys were found.

I didn't expect him to; afterall, no one drops a whole key ring of keys and doesn't hear it.

As it happens, I had just bought my house 1 month prior so all of my house keys were on my keychain, as well.

I'm simply sick, I want to cry but that wouldn't get me home or into my house. I had alerted the house supervisor who seemed to have a little bit of empathy for me. She called the Assistant Director of Nursing, while I stood there. *The ADON, unprofessional, weird and built like a BMW who didn't like anyone.*

As the manager told her of the events, I could vaguely make out that the ADON didn't care much about my situation. Why else would she ask "well who is the nurse?"

The manager said my name.

I could see the managers' facial expression change, a slight smirk came across her lips, but she quickly regained her professional composure.

It didn't miss me.

I know the look of someone who is trying to keep a straight face when someone says something inappropriate.

The house supervisor hung up the phone, looked at me and said that they would look into things.

I left the office, I was behind in my work, very behind.

I tried to catch up and clean up as best I could.

My night shift relief Nurse arrived.

She gave 2 shits, she was clearly irritated that I had missed giving some of the medications and that some things weren't done despite my telling her about the cna's stealing my keys and that I needed to search for keys, call insurance company, call tow truck, speak to supervisors. She seemed very annoyed.

Again, she could care less. Nurses ##ruthless

In the end, I took an Uber home, I tore out screening from one of my windows in the back and got the window open, fell on the floor and cursed all cna's ever to be created, showered, poured some wine and then cried.

I wasn't scheduled to work the next day, but I called off on Wednesday.

I stayed in the bed depressed all day Monday.

Pulled myself up and together on Tuesday. No call from any manager. I didn't expect one.

I coordinated a mobile locksmith to make new keys on site for my car, uber'd to my car, paid another locksmith for keys to the house, and then had the window repaired; about $400

Received not one call from a supervisor or anyone else in management.

Called on Thursday to quit my job. The staffing girl was very nice and she seemed genuinely concerned. How about we put you on the 3rd floor permanently and I'll talk to management for you.

The 3rd floor wasn't that bad and I did need my job considering I had just bought a new house.

Still no call from anyone in management regarding my stolen belongings.

The cna's on the 3rd floor were more professional and you didn't have too many problems with them.

The Nurses on that floor, well, that was different. They seemed to be okay with me until one of their favorite nurses who had gone part time decided to return to full time. Then they wanted me gone and well, that's pretty much what happened.

The Director of Nursing found a reason to fire Nechelle their staffing coordinator so that she could bring in one of her friends. (typical nursing stuff)

Once Nechelle was gone, the very next shift I came in to work they had scheduled me on the 2nd floor where they knew I wouldn't/couldn't work.

I told the manager that I could not work the 2nd floor. She told me that everyone had to take a turn and float.

I told her that my reason for not working on the 2nd floor had nothing to do with whether I wanted to float or not.

She told me that my situation had already been discussed with management.

I told her that I was refusing to work on the 2nd floor.

She called the ADON who said the same thing.

They wanted me gone and I knew it.

"you know that this is abandonement?" she said

I told the ADON that I had not accepted report or taken keys and that I would call and speak to the DON later.

"the Director of Nursing is already aware!"she said

At 7am she is already aware that I might call her. OK

I told them that I was going home, they told me that I would lose my job.

I said okay.

I walked to the elevator, Cam was sitting in the nurses station pretending to work on the schedule.

Because when they want you gone.........well.......

Sins of Nurses

"In three words I can sum up everything I've learned about life. It goes on."

-Robert Frost

CHAPTER 35

LEONARD

Leonard had been in a motorcycle accident about 12 months prior to coming to our facility. He was somewhere in his early 30's if I remember correctly. He had been living with his parents since his accident. I remember the day that he came to us from the mental health hospital, where he had been for the past week. He arrived in jeans, a t-shirt and a baseball cap. I was surprised that he looked so normal. Why did they bring him here, of all places? They said because we had the only "locked" unit in the area, which had an open bed for him.

Leonard was very polite, saying hello and smiling to everyone.

He constantly repeated himself, which was one of the first indicators that something wasn't quite right with him.

His family had tricked him to get him to the facility by telling him that he would be staying at the facility for just a day or two. Just until his parents could drive over and pick him up.

He seemed to be okay with that. His mother called that evening; I spoke to her at length. She cried most of the conversation. She felt a tremendous amount of guilt in having to place him in a facility. She told me that she and her husband had multiple medical problems and that they both felt that they were too old to deal with Leonard, they simply could not control him nor help him.

I could believe it, Leonard stood about 6'5 and appeared to be as strong as an ox.

I assured her that he was safe, although I knew that he wasn't.

This nursing home had a reputation as being one of the worst in the areas and it wasn't appropriate for Leonard. He needed to be in a facility geared toward helping persons with traumatic brain injuries, Not a nursing home.

There is a severe shortage of such facilities in this area and probably anywhere in the country.

From the time that Leonard arrived and got settled on the floor, he wreaked havoc in one way or another. When he was frustrated, he would push the other residents around and if he could, he would push the staff members.

Yes, physically push the staff and anyone else.

He could get pretty angry at times!!

He wandered around most of the day.

He looked just too normal for his own good.

If you didn't work there you could believe that he was a visitor.

Family members and new visitors would allow him to get into the code-locked elevator because of the way he looked. He spent most days looking for a way to get off of the unit and out of the building.

He would stand in front of the elevators waiting and hoping for a chance to get onto one of them. If he wasn't doing that, he would simply go from exit to exit trying to figure a way to get out and to go home.

When nothing worked and he became frustrated he would start to yell and punch things, he could be dangerous. We usually held him down and gave him a shot of Ativan when this happened.

AND when he wasn't exit seeking 'he was attempting to get into bed with one of the female residents. This drove us crazy.

We just weren't equipped to handle this type of patient in an Alzheimer's unit full of 80 year olds. We could barely manage the true Alzheimer's patients that we had.

Why couldn't we handle him?"

Well, for one elderly people could be redirected and given something to distract their mind. A game, an old TV show, even a sandwich. An Alzheimer's patient and a patient with an acute brain injury require 2 different types of care. They are two different types of people.

An acute brain injury happens overnight.

To make matters worst, Leonard's age was a factor; he was only in his 30's. He had just enough memory left to know that he wanted to go to the bar. That he wanted a drink. That he missed his mother and his father and that he didn't belong with all of these old people. *In his mind.*

We just weren't appropriate for him, this nursing home environment.

But then I had no control over any of this, I was just the nurse. I knew that this was to be another long day. I looked at the schedule, Robert was working this evening. More dread. I hated working with Robert, he had a drug problem and everyone knew of it. He would walk around singing and sweating. Everyone hated when he worked because although he was there, it was as if he wasn't. He was a lazy and useless waste of space when he worked. It was no secret that he smoked crack. More than one staff member had reported that he appeared to be under the influence of something at times.

Once, I had even reported that he and another CNA smoked marijuana when they were on their lunch breaks. I didn't see them but I could sure smell it on Robert when he returned.

The other CNA didn't work on my floor.

But when I spoke to management, I was told that just because I "thought" I smelled marijuana on him, this was not enough reason for the facility to act on this information. I was told that the facility could not test anyone for drugs based on the word of one person.

So let me get this straight I thought to myself. You hold me responsible for the lives of about 40 people. I'm responsible for their care, their medication, and even making sure that they eat. You trust that I would know how to handle things should an emergency happen, maybe someone will need CPR, a fire could break out and I have to lead and make critical decisions, monitor the health of my patients, BUT I cannot be trusted to know that a person appears to be under the influence of an illegal substance. That same person is responsible for caring for 10-15 persons.

However, this is the typical way that it goes. I'm over it. I'm used to it.

A week later, another nurse notices the same thing and then they decide to do a drug test on Robert.

But to show you how corrupt the system is, everybody knows there is going to be a drug test. The facility human resources female tells mostly everyone. It's their way of not losing staff. If they leak the fact that there is going to be drug testing tomorrow, anyone who might not be able to pass the test will have time to prepare for it. For instance, they could buy something to help them pass the test or use the famous "borrow urine" method from their girlfriend or boyfriend. Therefore, everyone knows that there is going to be a drug test today. As each person walks into the door, they randomly choose every other person to submit urine. So I'm in the room of one of the residents, I happen to look out of the window and I see Robert's car pull up in the parking lot. I head downstairs near the office where they are doing the testing only to see Megan the girl responsible for obtaining the urine samples (whom everyone knows smokes marijuana herself)approach Robert and take him into a back room for testing. He comes out in less than a minute and then leaves. I wait a few minutes to see where he is going. He gets into his car and leaves.

I go to the staffing girl and pretend as if I don't know that she has talked to him and I ask her why Robert hadn't reported to the floor.

She said that he had a family emergency and had to leave. Let me guess, he didn't get the memo that there was a drug test today. I looked at her

".... Idiot...." I thought.

I can't tolerate this kind of stupid shit. It became the joke of the facility. Her being responsible for the drug testing, especially when everyone knew she smoked marijuana herself.

I shook my head; she knew that the very point of the testing that day was to test HIM because of my accusations. A few days later, the urine results came in and three people were put on probation. Of course, Robert came back to work 2 days later; I'm sure, prepared to do his drug screen. He passed the drug screen. We all knew that he would pass with the advance notice and 2 days off to clear things up. We all knew that he had done something. He had actually told a few people. I think the story was something like he had brought his own urine from home, probably the urine of some friend.

I was pissed!!! It just wasn't fair; a nurse's job is hard enough without having to worry about the CNA being on drugs.

Robert seemed to walk around me with a smirk. He knew that I was probably the one who was trying to catch him. There was nothing that I could do. I guess you are asking yourself, "Self, what does any of this have to do with the story about Leonard?" Because at the end of this story you might be asking yourself, what kind of person would do this? I'm answering you in advance; I've just painted you a picture of the kind of person who could do this.

Back to Leonard standing in front of the elevator. Standing and walking from exit door to exit door trying to get out. Yelling and hitting. The facility elite (the unit managers, supervisors, director and even the administrator) knew that Leonard wasn't right for a nursing home Alzheimer's unit.

We all felt and knew that he was dangerous. It was easy to be intimidated by him. The female residents were terrified of him and rightly, so, he did much to terrify them. He was getting into bed with them and saying that they were his girlfriends.

All of the nurses felt helpless and this occurred every day that you worked.

The nurse to nurse report always revolved around Leonard and something that he had done.

The nurses tried everything to get him discharged permanently from our facility. No luck.

One evening he wandered into the room of Mrs. Shakir. He jumped into her bed and wouldn't get out. I heard her crying and yelling for help. I ran to her room. There he was, lying in her bed. I tried to convince him to get out of her bed. He wouldn't budge. I finally had to do something that I hated to do. I had to call Robert and ask him to help me. Robert came in along with the other nursing assistants. There were probably four of them and sometimes it took all of them to manage him.

Once his mind was set about something, changing it was very difficult.

It was probably going to take all of them to get Leonard out of that bed and out of that room. I left them and went down the hall to do some of my paperwork.

I expected to see them dragging him out of the room any second.

No one came out.

I heard an occasional loud laughter from down the hall.

Another loud laugh.

Eventually walked down the hall to see what was going on with Leonard and getting him out of the room. As I walked toward the end of the hall one of the nursing assistants, Jennifer, who I had grown to be friends with, grabbed my hand, hugged me and walked me in the other direction. She did this to keep me away from the room. She was laughing, "Don't go down there, you'll lose your license and we gone lose our jobs if you do." I looked at her.

"What?" I said

At that moment, I heard rustling sounds and then it sounded as if someone yelled for help.

I turned around just in time to see Leonard running down the hall. His face was "beet red." His lip was bleeding. He ran straight toward me.

He had an idea, I think, that I might be able to help him.

Robert was running behind him. I put my hand out toward Leonard to stop him and he did. He appeared out of breath.

"What's going on?" I asked Robert.

"Nothing! Nothing at all" he said as he turned and walked away. I turn to look at Leonard who was standing behind me.

"Are you okay Leonard?" He looked at me and said, "I'm fine, that motherfucker was trying to get me."

I then pulled his hand and began walking him toward his room.

"What happened?" He didn't answer me.

I had a feeling in my gut.

"You're safe." I whispered as I walked him to his room.

When I got to his room, I looked at his face. It was really red. His lip had a little crack in it, I cleaned it up. Otherwise, no marks, no scratches, no bruises, just his red face and cracked lip.

"What the hell happened? What did they do?"

I guess part of me already knew. *Should I call a manager*? Should I press the issue and see if one of the CNAs will admit to anything. They were all in on this.

I know this won't go well for me if I say anything.

It never has, it never does.

I looked at Leonard and helped him into bed. For a brief minute, he seemed completely normal. I think he saw the worry in my face.

"Don't worry, I'm fine." he said.

I looked at him and I said nothing. I stared at the wall. I told no one, I did nothing.

Sins of Nurses

"Non-black persons cannot possibly think that they may disrespect and mistreat 'black' people for over 150 years and that it will have no effect or bearing on their treatment when those same 'black' people have to care for them because they can no longer care for themselves and NO ONE IS WATCHING!"

-R.L Green

Chapter 36

BLACK AND WHITE

I would be telling you a lie if I didn't admit that there was a difference between black Nurses in a LTC facility and other races of Nurses. The difference is as wide and as deep as the culture of each race, like oceans. Just as there are differences in our lives, social statuses, conversations, the way we dance, raise our children, the way we speak, the things that are important to us, and even our credit scores. That difference does not stop when we enter the Nursing home and begin our workday. Other black nurses and CNA's will get this. Even nonblack nurses and CNA's who work with black nurses and cnas will get this. Other races will get it and agree in their heads because they can't say it aloud. Other races find it easy to work with black cna's and some black nurses because we continue to "cater" to those races. Somehow, we continue to think that white is better and that white is right. But then we've been brainwashed like that for a long time.

RACISM

Working with each other can be HELL. It makes you wonder (not me) why would white Nurses who could work in so many places choose to work in a dilapidated, dirty, old nursing home with ALL black people? Because their nice? Because they don't see color? I challenge that it is because they know how black people receive them. I realize that this is going to be a controversial statement but I'll say it anyway. It's because white people know that many blacks continue to place "white" on a pedestal. I see it all day long. If I walk into the nurses' station and there are other blacks there speaking unprofessionally, using profanity, breaking the rules. They will not stop. If the white Nurse walks into the Nurses' station they will respect her enough to stop. If I, as a black nurse make a comment as to this behavior I'm then viewed as a bitch who thinks that she is better than "US."

For some reason, I just can't want respect, I GUESS.

The same respect that you give my white counterparts. This is a form of Jim Crow that blacks can not move past. A nurse of any race other than black can get away with LOTS!! Black nurses are held to a different standard. A standard that must be excellent and perfect in Nursing. If my white counterpart makes a mistake, there is a hand tap and a "we understand" mentality.

If a black nurse makes the same mistake, it should be handled with a corrective action of some kind. She should speak to the Director of Nursing immediately to discuss this error and how this happened and how it should not happen again.

Here is an example; I worked the other day with Amber (a black nurse, like myself).

She and I were working the worst units in the building Hall 400 south and 400 north. The med pass is quite challenging, probably 10 accuchecks along with gtubes and other things that make it the worst hall in the building.

We manage to get through our rough dayshift .

Amber's shift is over. Mine is not, I'm working a double.

Amber's relief shows up.

It happens to be Meghan, one of the few white nurses working in this facility. She walks past us to the timeclock.

She eyes us but doesn't speak or acknowledge us. I've only seen her a few times and my encounters with her have usually been coordial. Not today........... *Ignore*

Amber is waiting down the hall at her nursing cart to give her report and to count. Meghan clocks and returns to the nurses station, sits down and starts to text on her phone. Completely ignoring Amber. Amber is watching her from down the hall. Still waiting.

The shift started at 3pm, it's 3:20p still not ready to count. Meghan is now busying herself with other things, shuffling papers, reading the 24hr reports, logging on to the computer; anything to keep Amber waiting.

There is a small incident unfolding. A resident is having a seizure. The day shift Supervisor is taking care of the resident and this incident and there are other nurses present. Meghan is standing by. I suppose she is standing by just in case they need her help or is it to annoy Amber? Clearly to annoy Amber, because the incident is taken care of and there are 2 nurses already there.

Amber asks Meghan about giving report and counting, she ignores her. I was a bit surprised. I mean, who flat out ignores another nurse like this? Everyone knows that Meghan has a problem with black nurses. At least black nurses who don't put her on a pedestal.

Anyway, it's now 3:35pm and Amber is still waiting for Meghan to take keys and receive report. Amber is trying her best to be professional and patient.

At one point I notice Meghan look over at Amber and continue to talk on her cell phone; it came across as very disrespectful. Eventually, Amber comes to me.

"I really have to leave, can you count with me?"

I really don't want to because I'm trying to stay on top of my own work.

"Sure."

As we are walking to the cart Amber says

"Meghan is really racist, you know that don't you."

"Yes, I've heard, but I haven't really had any encounters with her." I had heard this about her.

"watch her, you'll see it." Amber says.

"that bitch is lazy and she doesn't give out any of her medication, she puts on a good show like she does, but everyone knows that she doesn't medicate any residents that she takes care of…..watch her, you'll see."

"All of management seems to be blind to her. I guess it's because she's white."

"I'll have to watch her and see it for myself." I say to her.

We finish the count and report. She walks out of the door, she directly passes Meghan. Meghan doesn't say a word to her. As soon as Amber is gone, Meghan comes to me and asks for the keys.

"You want to count?" "Report?" I ask her.

"Nope, I'm good." She bounces away.

I walk away, I don't care. I have my own work to do. Down the hall I'm hustling trying to complete my accuchecks. It's getting late and I need to do this before the residents' have their supper.

It's now after 4p and they are due at 4pm. I look down the hall. Meghan is sitting at the desk talking.

I'm still hustling to get my accuchecks done.

Meghan's hall has far more work than mine.

Yet she is still sitting.

The supervisor returns to the floor. He sits at the desk and starts talking to Meghan. He's white.

Something is quite funny. They are both laughing really hard.

Its my opinion that if Meghan wore black he would wonder why she is still sitting and not doing any work at this very busy time. He doesn't "seem" to notice. They talk for a while.

It's 5pm and she still hasn't moved.

I notice that she looks down the hall and notices me watching her. She gets up and walks toward me saying that she is going to check on the other floors for a medication that she needs.

"ok."

I don't see her for a while. She still hasn't done any work.

One of the doctors comes in. She has returned and is sitting at the desk talking to him for a while. Eventually he leaves and goes to one of the other floors. She continues to sit at the desk. The supervisor is back. She sits and talks to him for a while longer. I glance at the clock it's 6pm. I'm struggling with my heavy med pass and thinking.

Amber was right.

The nursing assistants pass her left and right, nobody notices her not doing any work. One of the cna's stops and takes the time to play with her long blonde hair.

Again, If Meghan were black everyone would notice her sitting at the desk AND would be gossiping/complaining about her.

But they all know Meghan and no one is going to say a word.

Eventually I see her go down her hall for a while. It may have been 30 minutes later when I see one of her friends come to the floor to see her. They go outside for a smoke break. She returns later. I see her go down the hall with her cart for a short time.

It's now 8pm. She yells down the hall to me.

"I'm going on my dinner break." she leaves the facility.

I'm finally caught up on my work and sitting at the nurses station doing some charting. I guess I'll go on my dinner break when she returns. She is back in about 40 minutes but she keeps past the desk, doesn't say a word, and heads for the elevator. I wait for her to return. Not sure where she is. It's after 9pm I have to take my break, I leave.

I return. She is standing at the end of the hall laughing and talking with the supervisor. I walk toward the two. I need his help for something. As I'm walking toward her, I overhear her saying something to the effect of.........

"These nurses don't do their jobs."

"I don't think anyone has been medicated today."

" I don't think half of them give their medicine which is why we see some of the behaviors with the residents."

AMAZING! She is implying that Amber didn't medicate the residents on her shift earlier.

You who have barely passed any pills this entire shift, has a comment as to other nurses who don't pass medications.

WOW!

It appears that the Supervisor hasn't noticed a thing. Complete blinders on. How could she work the hardest unit in this building and not be busy? Have time to talk to him half the evening?

I know you are thinking, "but what makes this a race thing?" Trust me. It is and Meghan knows it as well. She knows that her implication of a black nurse not passing medications is very believable to another white person.

When she knows that she is guilty of not passing medication. Its' no secret that residents aren't getting medication. But who is not giving it? The black nurses or Meghan the only white nurse. It's no different than the racism that exists elsewhere. You know the racism where a black man and a white man commit the same crimes. The black man gets 40 years in prison without the possibility of parole and all the white people thinks that his crime fits the punishment. The white man gets 5 years, credit for time served and probation and it's a fair punishment for such a family man.

I have a question. (further controversy) There is a very high population of older white persons in nursing homes. Do you believe that some level of care may be in question by this generation of young, ignorant, lazy, cutting corners, minimal morals having, don't care about anything, subjected to daily incidents of racism by society, nursing assistants?

It's a very sincere question to ask yourself!

Two nursing assistants come out of a residents room as I walk by

" he better lay his white ass down, I'm not dealing with his shit this evening" says one of them.

"Niggers, you nigger bitches!" the resident yells.

They laugh and keep walking.

Sins of Nurses

"Don't be fooled by the glasses and what appears to be."

-Maxine N.

Chapter 37

SHAKIRA

Where do I begin? This day was no different than any other day. Receive report, give pertinent information to the cna's then start my day. Shakira is one of my cna's that I'm working with today, we've actually been working together for a couple of months. Everything has been going well. I've noticed a few things about her that I don't care for but overall she seems to be a decent cna. You don't have real high expectations of your cna's working at THIS facility.

I thought Shakira was a cna that had a slightly higher standard than the usual run of the mill cna.

We're a few hours into the shift and I'm looking for Shakira, I knock on one of the residents doors and then I simply enter. There is resident Kathryn lying on the floor wriggling from side to side. I look at Shakira who is standing there calmly making the bed

"what are you doing?"

"making the bed"

"but why is Ms. Kathryn on the floor like this?"

"she likes being on the floor"

I simply stare at her in disbelief. I move toward resident Kathryn and begin to move her to a sitting position.

"I need you to help me get her up"

"why? She likes being down there"

"I need you to help me, she can't be on the floor like this, you know that if someone sees this both of us will be out of a job"

She exclaims in irritation but comes over to help. She snatches her haphazardly and throws her on the bed.

"Be careful!"

"I don't care about her and you are beginning to get on my nerves!"

It's as I've been saying throughout this book , you have to pick and choose your battles.

Shakira just stares at me.

I had never seen this look before. She looked Evil. She wore glasses and an innocent looking school girl head band. At that moment there was nothing innocent or school girlish about her. She looked like the mean, uncaring, forty year old woman that she was. Everything inside of me wanted to report her actions but I knew that, per usual, it wouldn't matter. I turn to leave the room,

I hear Shakira.......

"uuughhh get your ugly ass over here!!"

At that moment she snatches resident Kathryn by the arm. Resident Kathryn slips from the bed and falls to the floor. Shakira didn't seem to have a caring bone in her body.

She stared at Kathryn as she lay on the floor wiggling from side to side.

I looked at Shakira's face.

She looked at me and in that moment, I knew that she truly didn't care.

Nothing inside of her cared about this woman, she didn't see a patient who she was to be helping. This was just work. A job to her.

I rush over to help, we pick her up from the floor and place her into the bed.

I look at Shakira, she's only complaining at having to bend her back to get her off the floor.

No emotion.

I assess Kathryn.

I walk out of the room, I can't do this today.

Later I start thinking about another Resident, Ms. Marlys who always has bruises on her body. Always bruises, arms ,chest, legs, everywhere. We've been testing her blood for any disorder which might account for all of the brusing. After watching Shakira, I really am starting to believe that she might be doing this.... but I can't prove it. You can never prove it. A suspicion in a nursing home means nothing more than paperwork. Paperwork that will be altered and amount to nothing. An investigation that will amount to nothing. Staff interviews that will amount to nothing. CNA'S like Shakira who go unchecked. She's been there for almost 20 years, they won't believe anything I say regarding her. Maybe if I wanted to talk about the new guy in the kitchen that she was sleeping with, maybe they'd listen to that. Her unprofessional, savage, ugly ways...they don't want to hear about, I said nothing.

****Sins of Nurses****

This book was completed. I was ready to send it for printing, and then there was the CoronaVirus. I found myself in its midst. I couldn't publish without adding at least one story.

Implement limited re-use of facemasks

"Facemasks should be carefully folded so that the outer surface is held inward and against itself to reduce contact with the outer surface during storage. The folded mask can be stored between uses in a clean sealable paper bag or breathable container."

CDC.GOV

BUT WE HAVE SUPPLIES?

Chapter 38

12 hours and the CoronaVirus

I arrived to my dayshift, scheduled via my agency. It was to be twelve hours. I'll manage. I had 25 patients that I would be responsible for. I received my report from another agency Nurse, minimal information. Of my 25 patients, 2 had scabies and 3 were possibly positive for the coronavirus.

Everyone stated that the possible coronavirus patients were not really positive, yep, everyone seemed pretty sure about that;

but we had to treat them as though they might be positive anyway. The story is that the three possible patients shared a four person room. There had been a fourth resident who had been sent out to the hospital a few days ago, I'm told he died a few hours after he had arrived. He had a fever and a cough. All of thestaff are stating that this fourth resident was a hospice patient who was actively dying.

This didn't matter to the hospital because no one could say with certainty that it was or was not covid-19.

Per CDC guidelines and the facility infection control nurse, the other 3 males in the room were to be quarantined until the results came back regarding whether the patient that had died was positive or negative for the coronavirus.

Then there were the other two residents who were actively being treated for scabies. They required isolation as well. This meant that every time I entered the room for care of any of these five residents I would have to gown, glove and mask!! Most of us nurses know that having one or even two patients on isolation is a pain in the ass but having 5 patients like this was going to be awful. I started my shift preparing to sanitize my cart *which I had started doing since the outbreak of the coronavirus.*

Many nurses and cna's were still not taking things seriously. I put on my gloves and began to look for disinfectant/bleach wipes to wipe my cart down. There are none on the cart. I asked the other nurse if she had disinfectant wipes, she stated that she had none.

What am I supposed to clean this cart with?

I look in the med room, the nurses station, treatment cart.....NONE! and I'm asking everyone, they all state that we don't have any. One person suggests that I go and speak to the guy in central supply. I locate central supply and there is a gentleman sitting in a makeshift office there. He looks up at me. I explain my situation. He states that the facility doesn't have the containers of bleach wipes. How is that possible with everything going on? How are nurses keeping the carts clean? I'm working with three suspected coronavirus patients and I need to frequently disinfect my cart. He stares at me as if I'm annoying him.

"I don't know what to tell you, we don't have anything."

He goes back to shuffling through his papers. I'm walking back to my cart. I'm ready to call my agency and leave. If I can't clean my cart how can I work and remain scabies/coronavirus free? I'm absolutely frustrated. Okay, I'll use hand sanitizer. Wait, no bottle of hand sanitizer. None anywhere, I look everywhere. I find a big bottle with about 1/8 th the amount in it. *There are also three wall hand sanitizers on my unit.* I go back to the central supply guy and I tell him that I have no hand sanitizer for my cart. He tells me that we are out and that I am going to have to use the wall station containers. I'm staring at him, he goes back to shuffling his paperwork. I head back to my cart. More frustration.

I have to be here for 12 hours, oh…11 hours now!

I see the housekeeper, she has a cart of supplies. I approach her and ask her what she is using to clean things with. Before she can answer I notice that she has a huge commercial container of disinfectant/bleach wipes and a disinfecting spray. I ask her if I can take some, she says ok. I grab a baggie from my cart and I start to rip off sheets of the disinfectant wipes from her container. She looks over and gives me a side eye as if to say "you're taking too many" I smile and take a few more. One problem solved.

Still haven't started my med pass.

I then go to the wall units and attempt to fill my empty bottle with hand sanitizer. IT'S FOAM!!

No filling my bottle. I get an idea, so I grab a cup from the med cart and fill it with foam hand sanitizer, I grab another cup and do the same thing. I'm creating hand sanitizer for my bottle that I will have readily available without running to one of the three stations on the wall of the hall that I'm working on. I have to let the foam sit for a while so that it will begin to liquefy. The joy of creativity in nursing.

I'm back to my medcart, taking everything off and wiping everything down. Ask me do I trust any nurse before me to have done this same thing so as not to spread any virus, germ, bacteria, or bug! NOPE! As I am wiping everything down one of my cna's approaches to tell me that the resident in room #14 wants to talk to me.

Uggggghhhhh, still haven't even gotten started. I go down the hall to room 14.

"Hello, i'm Nurse Green I'll be your nurse today, you needed to speak to me?"

"yessss, I've been telling the girls for over a week that I am itching like crazy and no one seems to be doing anything about it."

“okay, let me take a look, where is the itching?”

She shows me multiple suspicious looking areas….OH Shit, SCABIES!.......I back away slowly.

“I need to go and check somethings, I’ll be right back.”

I tell the cna to be careful because I’m sure that she has scabies. The cna responds that the men in the coronavirus quarantine room (which is right next door) have been complaining of itching as well.

CRAP!!

I go and grab the Unit Manager. Let’s get a second set of eyes on this. I go to her office and tell her of my findings and suspicions. She walks to the rooms with me to assess. She is in agreement that each person has scabies. That brings my infectious precaution number of patients to 7.

The two men who are known to have scabies.

Mrs. Bruce who has scabies and her room mate.

The three men next door who also might have coronavirus.

It’s only 8:30am, jeesh!

I go to the wall units to get foam sanitizer for my cups.

I have to go back and explain to the newly diagnosed five residents that they are all on isolation.

I gown, glove , mask and talk to the two female residents. They are fine, they just want treatment and for the itching to stop.

Gown, glove, mask …. Of course, there are no N-95 masks available. Just the surgical ones.

I think that I might have gone home if it were not for everyone assuring me that these 3 patients probably didn't really have the coronavirus.

My job right now is to tell them that they have scabies. Two of them have already been itching.

I'm standing at the entry to their room, room #10 and just as I am about to walk in, I hear the most loud, annoying thing that could possibly be heard right now.......and its stuck in my head

"CORONAVIRUSSSSS......CORONAVIRUSSSSS.....SHIT IS REALLLLL.....SHIT IS GETTIN REAL......thanks Cardi B

I go in and speak to the three patients. The third resident Mr. Boise is going to be a problem. He is a smoker and if you know anything about smokers in a nursing home, its that they are relentless about going outside during their smoke times. Mr. Boise immediately starts arguing with me about being confined to his room.

"I'm not going to do it!" "I'm no prisoner!"

I walk away.

I've said all that I'm going to say.

I've got to start passing my medications.

I'm at my medication cart passing medications and out walks Mr. Boise.

"Mr. Boise you need to go back into your room, you are on isolation."

"Try and stop me" as he keeps walking.

He thinks that he is going outside to smoke.

I'm following him, not touching him and keeping my distance as he walking past other residents without a mask.

Luckily the administrator, is nearby. She's been made aware of what is going on.

She demands that he go back to his room or that she will call the police.

He is yelling that he will call the police if we don't allow him outside to smoke.

She walks him back to his room.

He goes into his room and calls the police.

The police don't come. They call the facility to discuss options. They have been made aware that he has scabies and possibly coronavirus.

CORONAVIRUSSSS……CORONAVIRUSSSS…….UUGHH

He's in his room yelling and complaining. Out he comes again.

"Mr. Boise, please go back into your room."

He goes back into his room and appears to stay there for a while, I continue to pass medications.

I fill my cups with foam handsanitizer.I have a good amount of liquid to pour into my bottle.

I go to the room of my two original scabies residents. Two gentlemen who look as though they've come from under a bridge. Their room is absolutely disgusting. Its' cluttered and dirty.

I gown, glove and mask.

I go in to give them their medication. I can't wait to get out of there. Just as I am about to leave my foot slips a little. I look down to a medium sized brown wad on the floor.

Please tell me that this is not what it looks like I say out loud.

Both residents are alert. The resident in Bed A looks at me, he gets up and walks to the bathroom. I see the smears of feces on his sheets and bed rails.

NOOOOOOOOO!! No...... no .... no......

I finish giving the medication and step outside of the room. Immediately I'm squirting hand sanitizer on the bottom of my shoes. I double glove and start wiping the smears of poop from my shoe.

I have to focus on finishing the passing of the morning medication.

Here comes the unit manager with orders to start the treatment regimen on the new scabies patients.

She's pulled the medication for 3 of the patients from the Cubex/EDK and I can give their oral doses now.

The cream that is to be applied can be done by the night shift , she says.

I complain to her about the floor needing to be cleaned in room #11.

She says that she will let housekeeping know to take care of it. I go back to my medcart which is sitting near to Mrs. Bruce's room (the newly diagnosed scabies patient) in room #4.

"nurse do you know how long I will have to stay in my room?"

"should I call my sister?"

"how long before the itching stops?"

Before I can answer any of her questions, Mr. Boise sticks his head out of his room. I head toward him.

"Yes officer I need police assistance, I'm being held against my will." I hear him say.

I go to the Unit Manager. "Mr. Boise has called the police again. "

"You know what, he's going to have to go. I'm going to call his family and speak to the Director of Nursing."

Ok I say.

I head to Mr. Boises' room. Gown, gloves and mask. I explain to him that if he chooses to leave that it will be AMA. (against medical advice)He says that he understands and that he doesn't care. He wants out of here.

I step out of the room and the Unit Manager, Director of Nursing, and Administrator are there ready to speak to Mr. Boise.

They make it clear that he is leaving against medical advice and won't be allowed back to the facility. He doesn't care.

I gown, glove and mask to perform an accucheck (test the blood sugar) on Mrs. Bruce.

Once done there, I gown, glove and mask to perform an accucheck on Mr. Lock, the other newly diagnosed scabies patient. I have 4 blood sugars to check and a few more medications to give out.

Mr. Boise impatiently keeps sticking his head out of the door of his room.

"when will the police be here ? I want to get out of here!"

I ignore him.

I leave the unit to go outside for a quick 10 minute break. Wearing the mask non stop is stifling. I just want to step outside alone and take it off for a few minutes. I return a few minutes later and notice the housekeepers' cart outside of room #10. I see her step out for a second to grab something from her cart. She doesn't have on any protective gear. I get to the room. The door is closed, I knock and call to the housekeeper to please step out for a second. She says to give her one minute. I wait a few seconds. I call to her again.

"You have to come out now."

She finishes what she is doing and then steps out.

"Maam you can't be in that room without protection, you need to wear a gown, mask and gloves. That is why there is a sign on the door and the reason there are of those other things are on the door."

She apologizes and says that she was only in there for a second.

NOT TRUE, but whatever.

I think to myself, if those residents have coronavirus, so do you now, oh yeah, and you probably have scabies too.

I cannnnnttttttt!

I stand at my cart and click out medications and I do some charting. The CNA is passing ice and water to the residents. I notice that she is wearing the isolation gear but that she keeps it on for all of the rooms. I Shake my head.

"excuse me, are you not going to change your gown and gloves while you are passing water and ice?"

"why whats' the problem?"

"You're potentially spreading germs and scabies….."

She has an attitude and insubordinate demeanor.

I don't work here, I can't educate this staff.

I shake my head and walk away. I see the Unit Manager a short time later and tell her of the events. She appears equally frustrated. I end the conversation with the reality that is "the staff needs more education regarding PPE and the meaning of isolation . She agrees.

Back down the hall to my cart. I see the same housekeeper in the other isolation room. NO PPE!

I look at her and throw my hands up……I can't!!!

"I know, I know, I'll put it on right away"she says.

I walk away. Everyone is going to be infected at this rate.

I take my 30 minute lunch. It's 4pm. The police have arrived to pick up Mr. Boise.

I'm not sure where they are taking him. Probably to the local hospital. Hopefully it gets conveyed that he has scabies and possibly coronavirus.

Gown, glove, mask....., no gowns or masks......

I call central supply and tell the central supply guy that all of the rooms are out of gowns and masks. He arrives a short time later, looking slightly annoyed but he restocks the 3 rooms with the needed supplies.

Gown, glove, mask.....evening accucheck and medication for Mrs. Bruce. Back to the cart. Medication to the next room. A few more computer clicks as I go.

Gown, glove, mask....evening accucheck and medication for Mr. Lock. Back to the cart, medication to the next room.

Computer clicks as I continue to pass medications.

"Nurse, will you be bringing my pain medication soon?"

Yes, I'll be bringing all of your medication soon.

I get all of her medication.

"shit" she's out of her pain medication, her Percocet.

This is going to be a problem.

"Mrs. Jamison, I have all of your medicine except your Percocet it looks like you took the last one earlier."

I knew that I was giving the last pill on the card but I didn't think that it was the LAST card.....

"Hopefully its been ordered, I'll call the pharmacy and check for you." I tell her.

" ohhhh god what am I going to do without my pain medication?"

"are you sure that there is nothing there for me? My full name is Roberta L. Jamison.

"yes Maam ive looked and you're out."

"well can you give me Tylenol?"

I look at the computer and there is only one order for Tylenol to be given for an elevated temperature, for her.

"yes, here is some Tylenol."

I hand her two tablets and continue with my med pass.

I empty my trash, clean off the cart. Fresh water and ice. By the time I get to the desk and call the pharmacy. They tell me that she needs a new prescription and that they told us that 7 days ago.

"ok, thank you."

Its 6pm, I'm in a mad rush to finish my charting.

Treatments?? Not today.

Mrs. Jamison comes to the nurses station. Nurse you didn't do my bio freeze. I need that on my back, my knees , my legs and ankles.

I look at her.

Ok, just go to your room.

Pharmacy has arrived. I'm signing for lots of medication. All the creams are here to be applied for the 5 new scabies patients. No Percocet came in for Mrs. Jamison.

I go to sit down.

Jeesh I need to go to the bathroom.

Where is it?

Over 12 hours later and I haven't gone to the bathroom once today.

One of the cna's points me in the direction of the bathroom.

I return just as my relief is walking toward the desk. She is a few minutes late.

I immediately count with her. Give her a thorough report and leave. She looks depressed as to what her 12 hours is to hold.

Its 730pm, I get my time sheet signed. I head for the door.

****Sins of Nurses****

MORE…Sins of Nurses

I have a collection of stories that span 20 years. Book 2 to be released soon. In book 2 I intend to dwell a bit more on the aspect of racism in nursing and

CORRECTIONAL NURSING

Some of the stories in Book 2 will cover the things that happens in correctional facilities. Most people don't know that jails and prisons operate much like a hospital inside of a small town. Jails and prisons have units and floors that have a dental office, doctor office, clinic, and infirmary where much goes on. If you are seeing the dentist you may get your teeth pulled, filled or whatever thing that you may need. You can see the nurse about a rash, the std you never took the medicine for, the warts, the vaginal and penile discharges, the lump that's been on your breast for 2 years…you name it, when people get arrested they want it taken care of. People enter the jail with high blood pressure problems, heart problems, cancer, pregnancies, weird growths, even weird allergies. There are people who get themselves incarcerated so that they may be treated for a medical issue that they cannot afford to take care of on the outside. Many babies are born behind jail and prison walls every year. I worked at a jail where a female bragged that all five of her babies were born at the expense of the county jail. Some people come into the jail solely for medical treatment. I knew of an inmate who received all of his treatment for cancer by way of the county jail. The surgery and all of the aftercare involved. Others come into the jail and get treatment just because they know that it is available. If you only knew how many people that come into the jail knowing that they will be there only for a few days and demand that they get checkups, std (sexually transmitted disease) testing, dental exams and treatment before they are released back into society. From a medical perspective, this is the processing of an inmate. A person is arrested and brought to the jail where they are processed in. This processing is pretty much the same for males and females. All females are given a pregnancy test while there. Everyone is processed in the booking area and they cannot go into the jail until they have received clearance by the medical department. Every person will see the nurse. The nurse will ask a series of medical questions, take your vital signs, height and weight. Some of the questions may be concerning whether you take any medications, if so, what are they? When was the last time you took this medicine? Are you under the care of a physician? Are you pregnant? Do you have any medical problems that you are aware of? Any medical problems that you are aware that you have but aren't currently receiving treatment for? We then write down all of this information including any pharmacy information and/or physician information. All information is verified. If they have a diagnosis like HIV or high blood pressure but have not been taking any medicine and have not seen a doctor, they are put on the list to see the doctor on the next day that he comes in. In the meantime, a call will be made to receive orders. "Hello, Dr. Phelps, I have an inmate who has a blood pressure of 198/100, he says he takes Lisinopril but he hasn't taken it in about 5 months, he is also HIV + and has run out of his medicine and has not taken it in over 1 year. Neither the medical department nor the sheriff's department can afford to allow this person to simply go into jail, to a housing unit without proper medical attention. Why not? Because although they have been living on the streets for months not taking care of themselves and not taking any medicine, he or she might get to the housing unit and have a stroke, hit their head and die and then that family will say that the county, the sheriff's department, and the medical department are responsible. That we should have stabilized him or her before we processed them into the jail. Then there is that 2.6 million dollar lawsuit. All inmates regardless of whether they have neglected their medical care for 15 years or 15 days must be treated or treatment orders are being obtained while they are housed in the facility. All at taxpayers' expense. If that person is receiving an experimental cancer treating medication at $1400 a pill, the jail must continue that treatment. In some cases, a person who came into a jail under such a circumstance and it could be verified by the medical staff is going to be released. That is, brought before the judge as soon as possible, and they are going to do everything possible to get him or her released. Unless he killed someone. Trust me, they are going to get an emergency order to have him or her released rather than absorb such a cost. Other inmates will be processed normally, they will leave the booking or holding area and be sent within the jail. A nurse must administer medication to the inmates in the jail. That medicine could be high blood pressure medicine, diabetes, cholesterol, antibiotics, etc…There has to be a nurse for the jail that is connected to the courthouse. Mr. Womack gets 40 years for a drug charge, he thought he was going to be released but passes out. They will call for a nurse, you might have to run to the courthouse to administer some kind of aide. The dentist needs help. The doctor needs help. The psychiatrist needs help. The medical infirmary is housing ten inmates. Two pregnant females, three men who attempted to rob a convenience store-the van rolled over and caught fire, now they all have 2nd and 3rd degree burns which must be taken care of daily. One man had a cancerous mass removed from his neck…four are on suicide watch because they were given life prison sentences and they are suicidal. There are the inmates who have come to call the jail system their home away from home. So at 2am if they are coughing too much they will call a "medical emergency" and some officer is calling you to say "we need a nurse to come and check out an inmate who is having a heart attack." And then when you arrive the inmate who was having the heart attack says,

"I didn't mean I was having a heart attack, I said I couldn't stop coughing and it felt something like a heart attack. Could I have some cough syrup?"

You stare at him.

The officer is irritated and so are you. "Nurse Green I swear he said he was having a heart attack!!"

You bring him to medical and give him a couple of cough suppressants.

He is sitting in the medical unit looking smug. You are looking irritated. In the end we (nurses) have our ways with the smart asses who come to jail and want to play games. Oh we have our ways!

Sins of Nurses

A FEW WORDS TO KNOW

Adl's : (activities of daily living) the ability or inability to perform the things that we normally do, such as bathing, dressing, toileting, walking, grooming or feeding ourselves without assistance.

Administrator: (the leader or person in charge of the facility who is responsible for its operations, development, monitoring and direction of policies and procedures, and licensure. The Administrator has ultimate responsibility for operations with regard to staffing, payroll and benefits administration, in-service education, budget review and analysis and operational and capital expenditures. The incumbent researches and makes recommendations to the Board for personnel policy changes, salary increases, staffing increases, annual budget amendments, resident rate increases, outside contractual services, major capital improvements and grants.

Admission: The process/paperwork of admitting a person into a nursing home or hospital.

Alzheimers: Alzheimer's disease is a brain disease that slowly destroys memory and thinking skills and, eventually, the ability to carry out the simplest tasks. It begins slowly and gets worse over time. Currently, it has no cure.

Bedbound: A person, who is unable to get out of bed unassisted, may be confined to a bed or chair.

Bolus (gravity) feeding: Bolus feeding is an intermittent feeding most similar to eating a periodic meal. It would be like receiving a dose, then waiting a certain number of hours and taking another dose. Common methods of delivery for an intermittent dose may be to fill a large syringe or bag like container hooked up to the feeding tube and just letting it drain in over a short period of time. This is called bolus or gravity feeding. Bolus feeding is the practice of using a feeding tube to supply nutrition to individuals who cannot or will not eat by normal means. It is one form of a larger group of tube-feeding techniques collectively known as enteral feeding.

Census: Number of patients in the facility or a particular unit.

Charting Shift notations of what is happening with a particular patient, record of how they are doing, what they have eaten or drank.

CNA (certified nursing assistant): Assistant to the nurse, patient caregiver who assists with feedings, baths, and general care.

Continuous feeding: (Gravity-Drip Method) First, the formula will be poured into the feeding bag. The bag will be hung on a pole. The tube from the bag will be connected to the clamped feeding tube. Once the two tubes are connected, the feeding tube will be unclamped, allowing the formula to flow. As with the syringe method, gravity will move the formula through the tube. The flow can also be adjusted using a regulator clamp. When the feeding is done, a syringe filled with water will be used to flush the tube. Lastly, the tube will be capped and may be taped to your body. A resident might have several feedings during a day.

Pump Method: These steps are similar to the gravity-drip method. The difference is that the tubes are connected to an electronic pump. The pump will be programmed to deliver the formula at a set rate per hour. For example, with continuous feeding, you will slowly be fed throughout the day. If you need this approach, the feeding will be stopped every four hours. The tube will be flushed with water so that it does not get clogged. The pump method can also be used for bolus feedings.

Contracture: Contractures are essentially muscles or tendons that have remained too tight for too long, thus becoming shorter. Once they occur, they cannot be stretched or exercised away; they must be released with orthopedic surgery. Most of the physical therapy, occupational therapy, and other exercise regimens targeted towards people with spasticity focuses on trying to prevent contractures from happening in the first place.

Decubitus: Pressure ulcers, also known as decubitus ulcers or bedsores, are localized injuries to the skin and/or underlying tissue that usually occur over a bony prominence because of pressure, or pressure in combination with shear and/or friction.
Pressure ulcers occur due to pressure applied to soft tissue resulting in completely or partially obstructed blood flow to the soft tissue. Shear is also a cause, as it can pull on blood vessels that feed the skin. Pressure ulcers most commonly develop in persons who are not moving about or are confined to wheelchairs.

Dementia: Dementia is a broad category of brain diseases that cause long-term loss of the ability to think and reason clearly that is severe enough to affect a person's daily functioning. For the diagnosis to be present, it must be a change from how the person was previously. The most common form of dementia is Alzheimer's disease

Discharge: Release from a hospital or facility, may transfer elsewhere.

DON (director of nursing): Just as it implies…he or she is the Director of Nursing, and all disciplines underneath her. She answers to the Administrator.

INCIDENT REPORT: A facility report form that documents any illness, injury, incident, which occurs that, results in a near miss incident, hazard, injury or illness to a patient. It includes a detailed description of the incident and all involved personnel or witnesses. An investigation into the incident will be performed.

G-tube (gastrointestinal tube) or (feeding tube): A feeding tube is a medical device used to provide nutrition to patients who ... A gastric feeding tube (G-tube or "button") is a tube
Insert

JCAHO (Joint commission on Accreditation of Healthcare Organizations): It is an organization created to maintain the standards of quality of care in medical facilities in the United States. It is a nonprofit tax-exempt organization that accredits more than 20,000 health care organizations and programs in the United States. A majority of state governments recognize JCAHO as a condition of licensure and the receipt of Medicaid reimbursement.

Hospice: Hospice care is a type of care and philosophy of care that focuses on the palliation of a chronically ill, terminally ill or seriously ill patient's pain and symptoms, and attending to their emotional and spiritual needs.

LPN (Licensed Practical Nurse): A licensed practical nurse (LPN) in much of the United States and most Canadian provinces is a nurse who cares for people who are sick, injured, convalescent, or disabled under the direction of registered nurses and physicians. [1] In the U.S. states of California and Texas they are called licensed vocational nurse (LVN).

MAR (medication administration record): The book, which contains orders of prescribed medication for patients. Anything that the doctor has approved and that the patient may have, this includes anything from vitamins to narcotics.

Med cart or cart: Where the patient medications are cart and dispensed from, a mobile carting unit of medication.

MRSA (Methicillin-resistant Staphylococcus aureus) is a bacterium responsible for several difficult-to-treat infections in humans. It is also called oxacillin-resistant Staphylococcus aureus (ORSA). MRSA is any strain of Staphylococcus aureus that has developed, through the process of natural selection, resistance to beta-lactam antibiotics, which include the penicillins (methicillin, dicloxacillin, nafcillin, oxacillin, etc.) and the cephalosporins.

NP (Nurse Practioner): Practitioner (NP) is an advanced practice registered nurse (APRN) who has completed advanced coursework and clinical education beyond that required of the generalist registered nurse (RN) role. According to the International Council of Nurses, an NP/advanced practice registered nurse is "a registered nurse who has acquired the knowledge base, decision-making skills, and clinical competencies for expanded practice beyond that of an RN, the characteristics of which would be determined by the context in which he or she is credentialed to practice."[1]

NPO: Nothing by mouth (may be ice chips if approved by the doctor).

Pill call -passing meds- med pass: The process of giving medication to residents or patients.

POA (power of attorney): A power of attorney (POA) or letter of attorney is a written authorization to represent or act on another's behalf in private affairs, business, or some other legal matter, sometimes against the wishes of the other's. The person authorizing the other to act is the principal, grantor, or donor (of the power). The one authorized to act is the agent [1] or, in some common law jurisdictions, the attorney-in-fact (attorney for short). Formerly, a power referred to an instrument under seal while a letter was an instrument under hand, but today both are signed by the grantor, and therefore there is no difference between the two.

Pressure Ulcer: (bedsore) SEE DECUBITUS

Redirection: To change a pattern of thinking, change from one thing to another.

Report: A review of events from the ongoing nurse to the oncoming nurse as to what has happened during his or her shift.

Rn (registered nurse): A registered nurse (RN) is a nurse who has graduated from a nursing program at a college or university and has passed a national licensing exam to obtain a nursing license. [1]

Rounds: To walk from room to room to and to give report while laying eyes on each resident that they are discussing.

Station or nurses' station : Area where nursing and other entities gather to discuss residents or patients. You might find the doctors, therapists, managers, nurses and CNAs gathered here. Nurses will stop here to do paperwork or even drink coffee.

Sundown syndrome/sundowning: Sundowning is a psychological phenomenon associated with increased confusion and restlessness in patients with some form of dementia. Most commonly associated with Alzheimer's disease, but also found in those with mixed dementia, the term "sundowning" was coined due to the timing of the patient's confusion. For patients with sundowning syndrome, a multitude of behavioral problems begin to occur in the evening or while the sun is setting. [1][2][3] Sundowning seems to occur more frequently during the middle stages of Alzheimer's disease and mixed dementia. Patients are generally able to understand that this behavioral pattern is abnormal. Sundowning seems to subside with the progression of a patient's dementia. Research shows that 20-45% of Alzheimer's patients will experience some sort of sundowning confusion.

Telemetry unit: A telemetry unit is a unit in a hospital where patients are under continuous electronic monitoring. Telemetry, the practice of sending electronic signals from one place to another, is a tremendously useful tool in hospitals, as it allows hospital personnel to monitor heart rate, heart rhythm, breathing, and other things both by the patient's bed and at a remote location like a nursing station.

TOTAL CARE: A patient who must have all care performed for him or her. This care extends from bathing, feeding, dressing, toileting, turning, all care.

Trach or tracheostomy: Tracheotomy is a surgical procedure which consists of making an incision on the anterior aspect of the neck and opening a direct airway through an incision in the trachea (windpipe). The resulting stoma (hole), or tracheostomy, can serve independently as an airway or as a site for a tracheostomy tube to be inserted; this tube allows a person to breathe without the use of his or her nose or mouth.

Treatment(s): Any medical care that is ordered by the doctor which requires a skilled nurse. This could be cleaning a wound, changing a dressing, applying a medicated cream, professional tasks which cannot be performed by a CNA.

Treatment cart: The place where supplies are kept, to perform treatments. This is usually a mobile cart of supplies, creams, bandages, tape, scissors, saline, all of the necessary materials to perform a treatment.

Unit: The division of floors and halls based on skilled nursing factors…a unit may be a dementia or Alzheimers' unit, medicare bed unit, psychiatric unit….etc.

Unit manager/RCM: The immediate supervisor of the unit nurse.

Wound(s): A wound is a type of injury in which skin is torn, cut, or punctured (an open wound), or where blunt force trauma causes a contusion (a closed wound). In pathology, it specifically refers to a sharp injury which damages the dermis of the skin injury to living tissue caused by a cut, blow, or other impact, typically one in which the skin is cut or broken.

Wound care: The actual care of a wound that is performed by a nursing professional.

Sources*******`
Wikipedia.org
Mayoclinic.com
Google.com

Made in the USA
Monee, IL
19 October 2026

66036444R00213